Secrets of Success

Smart way to success for every student

Disclaimer: The information given in this book is presented for educational purposes only and is not intended to diagnose or prescribe for any medical or psychological condition, nor to prevent, treat, mitigate or cure cancer and the other diseases. This information is not intended to replace a one-on-one relationship with a doctor or qualified healthcare professional, but rather a sharing of knowledge and information based on research and experience.

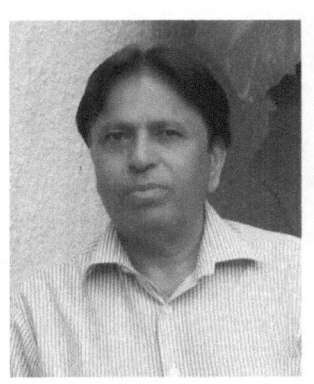

Written by
Dr. Om Verma
M.B.B.S., M.R.S.H. (London)
President,
Flax Awareness Society
7-B-43, Mahaveer Nagar III, Kota (Raj.)
http://memboy.blogspot.in
http://flaxindia.blogspot.in
+919460816360

Table of Contents

Flaxseed

Food for Body, beauty and Brain
Best tool for Personality Development

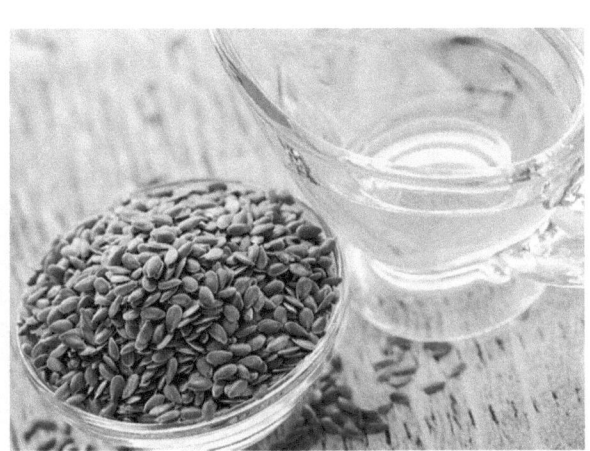

Secrets of Success

Normally people think that memory, intelligence or learning ability is a God gift and it is not possible to further improve or increase the brain powers. We take it for granted that it will remain as it is gifted to us by God. But the truth is just opposite. Understand that as you go to gym for workout to develop your six pack abs, feed your body with muscle building food and get sharp sculpted body shape. Friends, believe me if muscle can be built and remodeled, then why not your brain's hardware and circuit boards. If you feed your brain with proper food it needs, follow simple instructions and take advantage of neurobics or mnemonics, you can immensely increase your brain's abilities.

We have tremendous powers locked inside our brains, but we are not using them to full extent. Dr. William James, considered the father of modern psychology, pointed out that "the average human being uses only 10 percent of his mental capacity." We still have to find out how much power or secrets are hidden in our brain.

Nowadays scientists have discovered mysterious techniques and nutrients to boost our brain powers. Today I shall raise curtains from all these secrets; I shall disclose all hidden tricks and tips. Today you are going to learn how your CPU; the brain tightly packed in a bony cabinet, functions. I teach you how each component and microprocessors works and how the best insulation material can be prepared. I also disclose the right technique to sharpen your brain and to make you an intelligent and successful scholar.

Today you will learn how to crack every examination you face, solve every question, defeat every opponent and get highest possible marks. You are going to write new equation of education and success.

Friends new boundaries and horizon of success is ready to welcome you. Today we shall discuss in detail about some great nutrients and supplements to boost your memory, learning, imagination, creativity and concentration. If you follow our suggestions and apply simple tricks you achieve a successful personality. This short e-book is going to prove a turning point in your life. Wish you luck.

Visit us at http://memboy.blogspot.in

Science of memory

Memories are the internal mental records that we maintain, which give us instant access to our personal past, complete with all of the facts that we know and the skills that we have cultivated. The following are primary stages of the human memory process.

- Encoding
- Storage
- Retrieval
- Forgetting may constitute the fourth stage of memory, although forgetting is technically a breach in memory retrieval.

During the encoding stage, information is sent to the brain, where it is dissected into its most significant composing elements. Some group of brain cells processes incoming stimuli and translates that information into a specialized neural code. In the storage stage of memory formation, the brain must retain encoded data over extended periods of time. Retrieval stage constitutes the right of entry into the infinite world of stored information, where we bring old information out of permanent memory back into working memory, which can be mentally manipulated for usage.

Science of Memory

Learning is an active process that involves sensory input to the brain, which occurs automatically, and an ability to extract meaning from sensory input by paying attention to it long enough to reach working (short-term) memory, where consideration for transfer into permanent (long-term) memory takes place.

Vision has a much longer history in the human experience than does the printed word. By exploiting this competency, students learn quickly when they can visualize the concept while studying, by directed use of the mind's eye, where mental pictures can be developed.

Writing words in the air on an imaginary blackboard forces students not only to visualize the order of letters in a word, but to maintain visually what they have already written in working memory as they continue to write. When young learners are taught to construct diagrams that show relationships, their memory of content improves substantially.

Once the elements that make up an experience are classified according to their special patterns, each part is shunted to a different brain region for further detailed analysis. The various pieces of new information get stored in neural circuits distributed throughout the cerebral cortex. Because the elements making up a memory reside in multiple cortical areas, the stronger the network linking the associated pieces together, the more resistant to it will be to forgetting.

As the brain transacts learning events, physical changes occur both within brain circuitry and in its structure-function correlations. Memory is quite fluid, and, over time, the brain continues to revisit and reorganize stored information with each subsequent experience, reprogramming its contents through a repetitive updating procedure known as brain plasticity. This is advantageous, since improvements are made repeatedly to existing data. Prior knowledge is revised based on new input, resulting in a more accurate representation of the current world, increasing one's probability of thriving.

The relationship between learning and memory

While memory cannot occur without learning, once information has been learned, our memory may allow the learning to decay. Stress and multitasking are among the chief causes of memory lapses. Memory failure most likely reflects the consequences of stress, poor nutrition and exhaustion.

Emotions

Emotions can act as an enzyme to learning. In school, mere exposure to content information (lecture, text, etc.) is no guarantee that it will reach the personal/emotional threshold of "personal importance" to the learner, where encoding the information for permanent memory storage is deemed warranted. What students encode depends on what they are paying attention to at the time. Although we often wonder why our students forget important lesson content, the bigger problem is, was it ever encoded for memory?

Hippocampus – Memory Chip in the brain

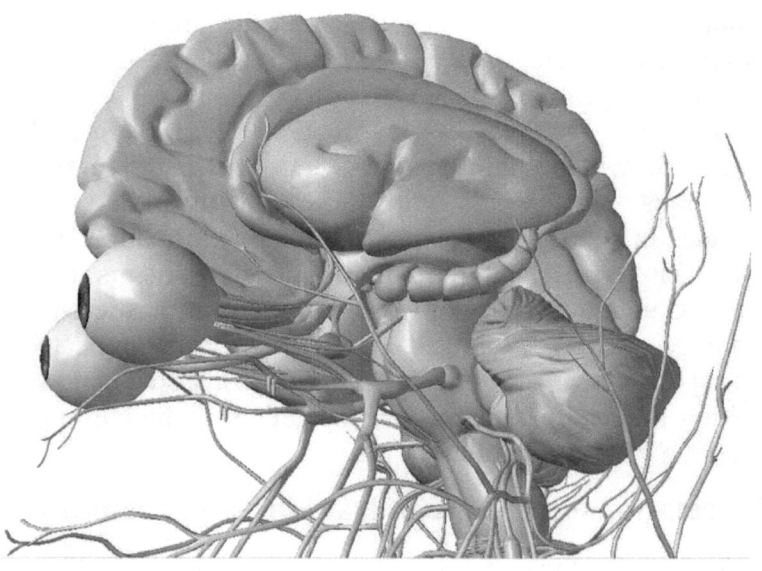

Several connected brain regions play key roles in memory formation, including the thalamus, amygdala, hippocampus and cerebral cortex. It is the interaction of nearly all parts of the brain that allows for the construction of our memories.

The hippocampus plays a crucial role in forming and storing our memories of facts and events. Initially, short-term memories (or random access memory) are briefly stored in the hippocampus, prior to being transferred to other brain regions where they are consolidated with prior knowledge into long-term memories (Hard drive storage). While persistent stress can damage hippocampus brain cells, patterns, emotions, relevance, context, content and sense-making boost attention, memory formation and recall. Collectively, they can determine what information reaches permanent memory storage. As Stanford Erickson summarized the requisite emotional element in learning, "Students learn what they care about and remember what they understand."

When information is determined to have potential long-term value, the hippocampus links the significant elements of that event or experience together, forming a permanent memory. Brain-imaging studies have shown heightened activations in the hippocampus not only when we are recalling memories but also when we put the mind on "wander and wonder." This has important implications concerning creativity and innovation, which are based on our ability to manipulate and expand on stored factual information.

Emotional experiences (both positive and negative) enjoy the highest probability of reaching permanent memory storage. It is the amygdala-hippocampus connection that fosters the development of our most memorable moments in life. In the classroom, emotions determine what students pay attention to, which impacts what students will later remember.

Mnemonics help

When attempting to memorize unrelated terms, mnemonics present the most practical solution. For students attempting to remember the most important neurotransmitters, the term "San Dope" works effectively.

- Serotonin 5-Hydroxytryptamine

- Acetylcholine
- Norepinephrine
- Dopamine
- Oxytocin
- Phenylethanolamine
- Epinephrine (adrenaline)

Prime Minister of Memory - Alpha-Linolenic Acid ALA

Alpha-Linolenic acid (ALA) is an essential omega-3 fatty acid found in seeds (china and flaxseed), nuts (notably walnuts). This is Prime Minister of omega-3 community. Other omega-3 fats such as DHA and EPA are grand children of ALA and nor considered essential.

Alpha-Linolenic Acid (ALA)

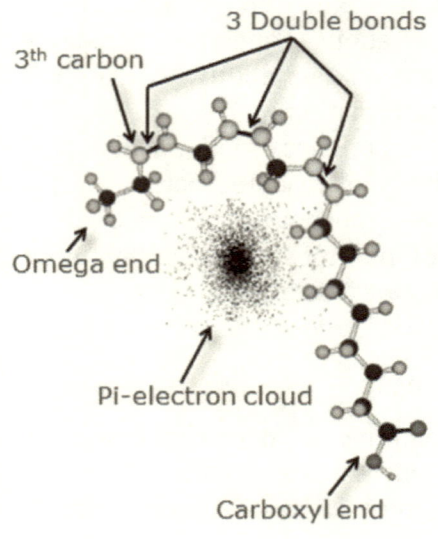

- Short Formula   18:3 n-3
- That means it has a chain of 18 carbons, 3 sis double bonds and first double bond is located after 3rd carbon from omega end.
- Melting point -11 degree Celsius

Docosahexaenoic acid DHA

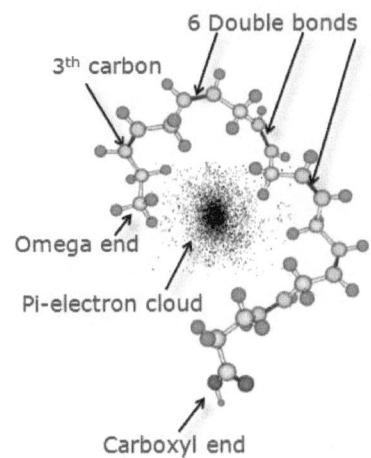

Docosahexanoic acid DHA

6 Double bonds

3th carbon

Omega end

Pi-electron cloud

Carboxyl end

- Short Formula   22:6 n-3
- That means it has a chain of 22 carbons, 6 sis double bonds and first double bond is located after 3rd carbon as usual.
- Melting point -50 degree Celsius

Eicosapentaenoic acid EPA

- Short Formula   20:5 n-3
- That means it has a chain of 20 carbons, 5 sis double bonds and first double bond is located after 3rd carbon as usual.
- Melting point -56 degree Celsius

Dietary source of EPA and DHA

Cold water fish and shellfish - salmon, sardines, mackerel, herring, and tuna.

Functions of omega-3

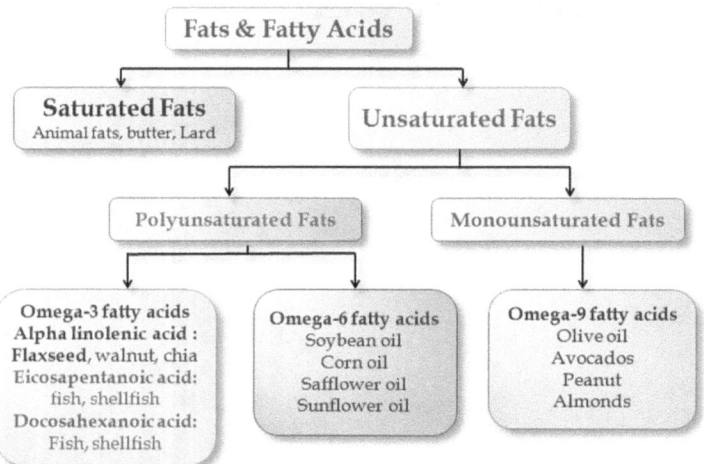

- Anti-clotting (thrombolytic) effect – acts as Natural Aspirin.
- Lowering the risk of heart disease – heart attack (Coronary Artery Disease) and atherosclerosis.
- Lowering triglycerides in the blood.
- Lowering high blood pressure.
- Reduction in heart irregularities – Arrhythmia.
- Helping to alleviate mood disorders, such as depression. Reducing aggression
- Helping patients with attention deficit/hyperactivity disorder (ADHD), dyslexia and dyspraxia
- Helping to improve memory and learning skills, and prevent Alzheimer's disease
- Improves immunity and Alleviates allergic disorders

8

- Improving inflammatory skin disorders such as psoriasis and eczema.
- Alleviating osteoarthritis, gout and rheumatoid arthritis (RA).
- Alleviating Pre Menstrual Syndrome PMS.
- Alleviating Menopausal Symptoms – Hot flushes, dry vagina, mood swing.
- Improvement of vision.

Arachidonic Acid AA

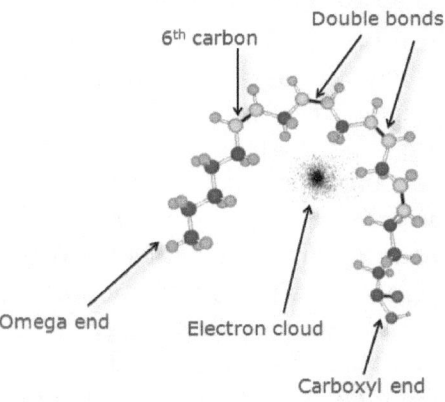

- Short Formula   20:4 n-6
- That means it has a chain of 20 carbons, 4 sis double bonds and first double bond is located after 6th carbon from omega end.
- Food sources - butter, animal fats, especially pork, organ meats, eggs and seaweed.

Omega-3 increase membrane fluidity

The brain has a huge number of cell membranes which are made up of fat. The fat make up of the brain is a little different than the rest of the body - only PUFAs allowed into the healthy brain in any appreciable amount are the ALA omega 3 derived

DHA (a long-chain omega 3 fatty acid) and the LA omega 6 derived arachidonic acid (AA). In addition, while AA is found in equal amounts all over the brain, DHA is found predominately in the gray matter. That's where our thinking takes place.

Let me explain a bit about the actual structure of these molecules. Saturated fats make rather tough and hard cell membranes all on their own. Their structure is pretty straight and tough, and they make cell membranes that look like this:

iiiiiiiiiiiiiiiiiiiiiiiiiiiiiiiiiiiiiiiiiiiiiiiiiiiiiiiiiiiiii

PUFAs have unsaturated double bonds, which make them bend and become weaker at double bonds. Cell membrane made of PUFAs that look like this:

iiiiiiLiiiiiiiiiiLiiiiiiiiiLiiiiiLiiiiiiiiiiiiiLiiiiiiiii

You can see that the unsaturated double bonds break up the structure a bit, and Dr. Paul Jaminet call this **"increasing membrane fluidity."** Important cell membrane proteins, such as ion channels, depend on the presence of PUFAs to be incorporated correctly into the membrane. If all is well, the PUFAs serve as part of "lipid rafts" that are required for transport of protein and signals through the membranes, the formation of synapses, and maintaining the integrity of the neuronal membranes. All of these functions are dependent upon omega-3 fats and are important and vital for the brilliant functioning of our complex brains.

Dr. Paul had nicely represented the role of PUFAs in neuronal cell membranes by simple "L" and "i" drawing of the cell membrane:

Omega 3 fats - especially DHA - are unique mainly in that they don't possess any real shape. They have so many double bonds that can twist and bend so easily, they change the shape very rapidly and under the slightest pressure fold up into tiny balls or slip out of the way. This is what makes salmon oil so slippery, especially at body temperature.

So a omega-3 rich membrane is barely a membrane at all. Rather a unique soap bubble like structure. A biological e x t r e m e. We don't even have a suitable letter in the alphabets for it;

even M has only three bends. DHA has six double bonds. This is what human intelligent brain depends on.

We can make sufficient DHA from ALA omega 3 fat found in flaxseed, if we have niacin, vit B-6, vit-C, magnesium and zinc in our body. We have enough evidence that if you consume flaxseeds regularly, your body makes sufficient DHA required for a high end brain.

The omega 6 derived AA is also important in the brain - it initiates and controls the inflammatory response, which is a critical function. The ratio of omega-3 and omega-6 is also very important, most ideal being 1:4. We can also make sufficient AA from LA omega 6 found in flaxseed, if we have niacin, vit B-6, vit-C, magnesium and zinc in our body.

Cis and Trans configuration

The two carbon atoms in the chain that are bound next to either side of the double bond can occur in a cis or trans configuration.

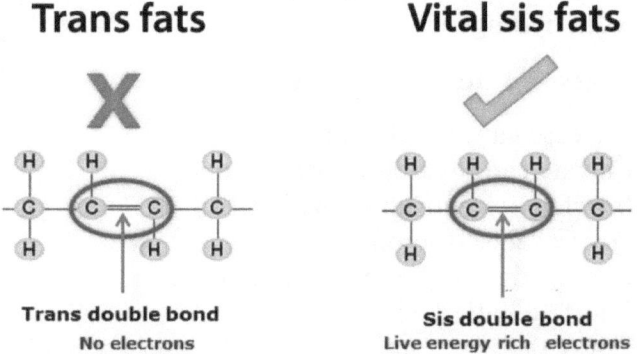

Cis configuration

- Cis configuration means that adjacent hydrogen atoms are on the same side of the double bond.

- The cis configuration causes the chain to bend by 35 degrees and cis fatty acids are thermodynamically less stable than the trans forms.
- The cis fatty acids have lower melting points than the trans fatty acids or their saturated counterparts.
- Cis fats have live, energy rich electrons
- Sis fats are rich in live, energy rich electrons.
- Electrons are key to health and longevity. This is biggest "Anti-entropy Factor".
- Electrons are extremely important to the body's overall energy exchange potential "the flow of life force."

Trans configuration

- A trans configuration, by contrast, means that the next two hydrogen atoms are bound to opposite sides of the double bond.
- As a result, they do not cause the chain to bend, and their shape is similar to straight saturated fatty acids.
- Most fatty acids in the trans configuration (trans fats) are not found in nature and are the result of human processing (e.g., hydrogenation).

Trans Fats – The deadly fats

- Increase cancer risk factors.
- Elevate cardiovascular risk factors.
- Interfere with insulin function.
- Decrease testosterone.
- Change the fluidity of cell membranes.
- Interfere with the healing fats.
- Trans fats are "anti-human", electron-poor, directed into the past, life functions are paralyzed, lacks energy and strength because the electrons that are in harmony with the sun as "life-element" are missing.
- Trans fat is the biggest enemy of mankind.

Prostaglandins - Overview

- Localized tissue hormones.
- They do not travel in the blood like hormones.
- Prostaglandins are potent but have a short life and are either locally active (Paracrine) or act on the same cell (Autocrine) within which they are synthesized.
- The prostaglandins perform different functions in the body.

Good and Bad Prostaglandins

Good – Anti-inflammatory
   o Series 3 prostaglandins
   o Series 1 prostaglandins
Bad – Pro-inflammatory
   o Series 2 prostaglandins

Good Prostaglandins	Bad Prostaglandins
Decreased platelet aggregation (prevents blood clotting)	Increased platelet aggregation (helps in blood clotting)
Vasodilatation (widening of blood vessels)	Vasoconstriction (narrowing of vessels)
Anti-inflammatory effect	Pro-inflammatory effect
Immune system enhancement	Immune system suppression
Increased oxygen flow	Decreased oxygen flow
Decreased cell proliferation	Increased cell proliferation
Decreased pain	Increased pain
Widening of respiratory passages	Narrowing of respiratory passages
Increased endurance	Lowered endurance

Prostaglandins - Functions

- Cause constriction or dilatation of blood vessels.
- Cause aggregation or disaggregation of platelets.
- Sensitize spinal neurons to pain.
- Constrict smooth muscle.
- Regulate inflammatory mediation.
- Regulate movement of calcium and other minerals & nutrients in the cell.
- Control hormone regulation.
- Control cell growth.
- Regulates cellular communication.

Series 3 prostaglandins

- The Series 3 prostaglandins are formed at a slower rate and work to attenuate excessive Series 2 production. Their response is "less vigorous".
- The omega-3 pathway might therefore be likened to the "slow lane".
- Adequate production of the Series 3 prostaglandins seems to protect against heart attack and stroke as well as certain inflammatory diseases like arthritis, lupus and asthma.

Series 1 prostaglandins

- Series 1 prostaglandins are Anti-inflammatory, Thrombolytic - Decreased platelet aggregation (blood clotting), pain reliever and control cellular activities.
- The strong anti-inflammatory properties help the body recover from injury by reducing pain, swelling and redness.

Series 2 prostaglandins

- Series 2 PG seem to be involved in swelling, inflammation, clotting and dilation.
- Series 2 prostaglandins are "fast lane" i.e. involved in intense actions and play a role in swelling and inflammation at sites of injury. This is not at all a "bad"

14

effect, but an important protective mechanism - the body's way of immobilizing the affected site to prevent further injury and facilitate healing.

- Series 2 prostaglandins also seem to play a role in inducing birth, in regulating temperature, in lowering blood pressure, and in the regulation of platelet aggregation and clotting.

Omega-6 / Omega-3 Metabolic Pathways

Although most omega-3 and omega-6 fatty acids are generally referred to as "essential" fatty acids, only linoleic acid (LA) of the omega-6 family and alpha-linolenic acid (ALA) of the omega-3 family are truly "essential". Once we have either LA or ALA, our body has enzymes that can convert these fatty acids into all the other different types of omega-6 and omega-3 fatty acids.

Omega-6 / Omega-3 Metabolic Pathways

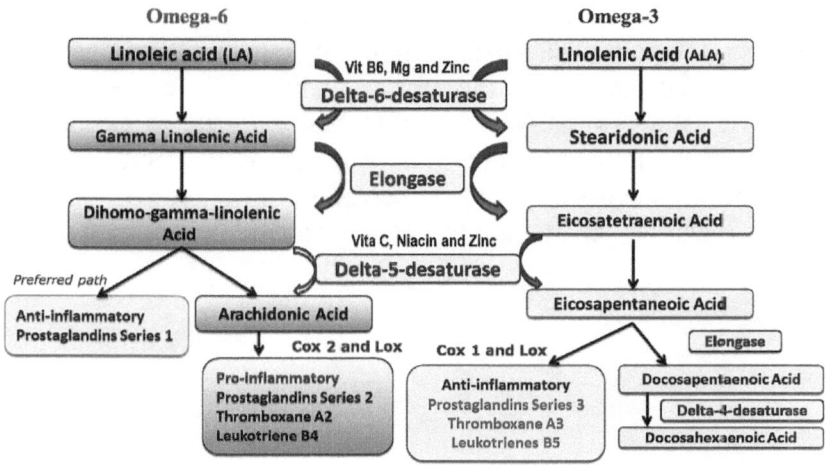

Prepared by Dr. O.P.Verma

It turns out that both the omega-3 and omega-6 pathway utilize the same enzymes, and both omega-6 and omega-3 fatty

15

acids have to compete for these enzymes in order to produce their final product. Studies have reported that the enzymes used in these pathways were found to prefer the omega-3 pathway. It turns out then that in diets high in omega-3 fatty acids, most of the enzymes will be "busy" converting the omega-3 acids.

The omega-6 fatty acids, Dihommogamma-Linoleic Acid (DGLA)) in particular, can be converted to either the anti-inflammatory PG1 or into arachidonic acid (AA), a precursor of PG2. Conversion of DGLA into PG1 does not require any enzymes, but conversion of DGLA into AA requires the enzyme delta-5 desaturase. In diets high in omega-3, most of the delta-5 desaturase will be used in the omega-3 pathway; few delta-5 desaturase will be available to convert DGLA into arachidonic acid, and subsequently, PG2. DGLA ends up being converted into the anti-inflammatory PG1 and inflammation is therefore decreased.

In a diet low in omega-3 fatty acids, large quantities of delta-5 desaturase enzymes are available to convert DGLA into AA. The available AA is then converted into the inflammatory PG2. Thus, the more omega-3 fatty acids present in our body, the fewer enzymes are available for converting omega-6 fatty acids into the inflammatory prostaglandins. A balance of omega-6 and omega-3 fatty acids is therefore essential for proper health. However, the typical Western diet has evolved to be high in omega-6 and low in omega-3 fatty acids. While omega-6 fatty acids are not necessarily bad, a skewed ratio in favor of too much omega-6 can be detrimental to one's health.

Balanced N-6/N-3 ratio – road to health, Ultra wellness & longevity

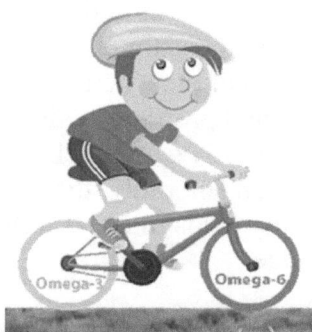

Road to health & longevity...

Both groups of prostaglandins perform vitally important functions and supplement each other through complex and multi-faceted interactions. For centuries ratio of Omega-6 and Omega-3 was perfect e.g. 2:1 or even 4:1 (very ideal ratio).

N-6/N-3 ratio out of balance - road to aging, disease & death

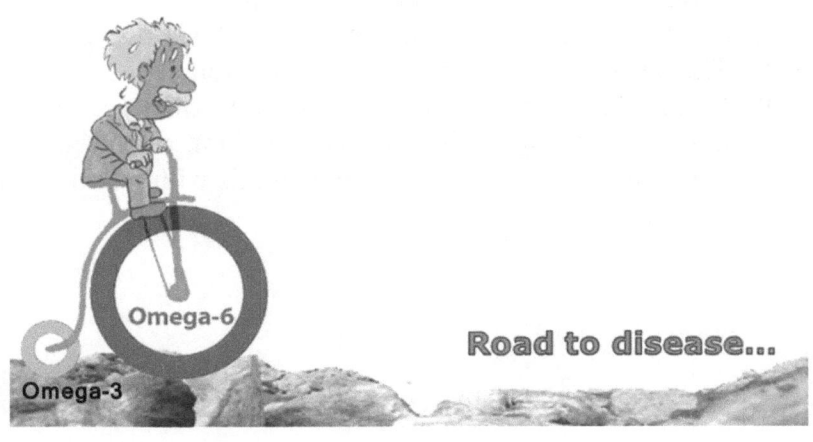

Road to disease...

17

But after the global switch to industrial agriculture and processed foods it is 20:1 or more (!!!).

- This throws the body into the state of chronic inflammation, giving rise to a whole array of clot and inflammation-related chronic diseases, including thrombosis, arthritis, diabetes, atherosclerosis and coronary heart disease (CHD, cancer and asthma.
- There is only one crucial condition that must be fulfilled if the entire system is to work well and promote health, rather than disease. This condition is B A L A N C E.
- For the prostaglandin pathways to run smoothly, the intake of omega-3 and omega-6 fatty acids must be well-balanced, within the 1:2 to 4:1 range.

Risk of eating fish

- Fish is Contaminated with deadly poisons like mercury, dioxins, polychlorinated biphenyls (PCBs), and pesticide residues.
- Very high levels of mercury can damage nerves in adults and disrupt development of the brain.

Benefits of eating flaxseed

- Flaxseed has much more Omega-3 than fish. Flaxseed had Alpha-linolenic acid, which is essential fatty acid and has ability to make all other omega-3's our body needs.
- There is no risk of mercury contamination.
- Flaxseed also provides us lot of fabulous fiber, legend lignans, and magic minerals like selenium, zinc, Mg, potassium and vitamins. You get all this without killing a creature.

Flaxseed - Omega-3 Fats

Building Block of Brain and memory

Omega-3 Fats- Reversing Many Aspects of Neurologic Aging

The cardio protective power of omega-3 fatty acids has been thoroughly documented in clinical literature. Less well known is their paramount role in optimizing many facets of brain function, from depression, cognition, and memory to mental health.

Recent research has opened up a new horizon in our understanding of omega-3s' profound ability to halt age-related decline and pathology, shattering the long-held medical belief that brain shrinkage and nerve cell death is progressive and irreversible. Omega-3s have been shown to possess antidepressant and neuroprotective properties.

Omega-3 - Key Nutrient from Cradle to Grave

Approximately 8% of the brain's weight is comprised of omega-3 fatty acids—the building block for an estimated 100 billion neurons. They play a host of vital roles in neuronal structure and function, protecting them from oxidative damage, inflammation, and the cumulative destruction inflicted by other chronic insults.

Embedded in the omega-3-rich neuronal membrane are numerous proteins and complex molecules required for electrochemical transmission and signal reception. Scientists have recently shown that the precise balance of fatty acids in brain cells helps determine whether a given nerve cell will be protected against injury or inflammation, or whether it will instead succumb to the injury.

Omega-3s accumulate in the human brain during fetal development. The amount of the omega-3 has been closely tied to intelligence and cognitive performance in infancy and childhood. Early developmental deficits in brain content of omega-3s have been associated with poor brain maturation and neurocognitive dysfunction. These are manifested especially in the area of attention, increasing the risk for attention-deficit/hyperactivity disorder (ADHD) and other behavioral disturbances. Later in life, declining levels of Omega-3 fats may contribute to development of aggression, anxiety, depression, schizophrenia, dementia, and a variety of other mental health and even criminal conditions.

Scientists are having great success at reversing many of the fundamental age-related decreases in brain function correlated with omega-3 deficiency. ADHD and related conditions can be prevented or mitigated by supplementing infants and nursing mothers with Omega-3. A remarkable animal study has just revealed that omega-3 fatty acids halt the age-related loss of brain cell receptors vital to memory production, and show potential for increasing neuronal growth.

Omega-3 - A Natural Crime Cutter?

Recent findings suggest that some criminal and aggressive behaviors are closely correlated with low serum omega-3 levels, which are linked to lower levels of honesty, and self-discipline. These effects may be related to alterations in serotonin turnover, which controls impulsivity and aggression-hostility behaviors.

There is a solid data indicating that optimal omega-3 intake at all ages is a promising avenue for subduing aggression and hostility. For example, omega-3 supplementation in autistic children with severe tantrums, aggression, or self-injurious behavior produced significant improvements compared with placebo, without adverse effects. And stressed but otherwise healthy volunteers given Omega-3 Fats reported a significantly improved rate of stress reduction, suggesting an adaptogenic role for omega-3s (adaptogens help the body respond to imposed stress in a variety of ways).

In a group of drug abusers, supplementation with Omega-3 Fats 3 months produced significant decreases in anger and anxiety scores compared to placebo recipients. Similarly, in young adult prison inmates, multi-supplements featuring omega-3s produced significant reductions in antisocial, violent, aggressive, and transgressive (rule-breaking) behavior.

Omega-3 – Cures Cognitive Decline and Memory Disorders

Omega-3 intake is strongly associated with many different measures of cognition and memory in numerous studies, and there's compelling evidence for potent neuroprotection over long time periods. Insufficient omega-3 intake is strongly correlated with diminished adaptability of brain synapses and impaired learning and memory. People with lower omega-3 levels may be more likely to suffer from a host of cognitive impairments including dyslexia, ADHD, and cognitive decline.

Laboratory studies shed light on these observations, suggesting that omega-3 supplementation may enhance brain function through increased production of the membrane-rich neurites required for new synapse formation. Other protective and cognition-enhancing effects include improved neuronal cell membrane characteristics resulting in enhanced neurotransmission, increased synaptic release of vital neurotransmitters such as serotonin, and neuroprotection from inflammation and oxidant-related damage including those induced by antipsychotic medications.

In healthy adults, increased omega-3 intake is positively associated with greater brain volume in regions associated with emotional arousal and regulation of behavior. People who get more omega-3s have bigger, more functional brains.

Flaxseed is called SIM CARD of Mind

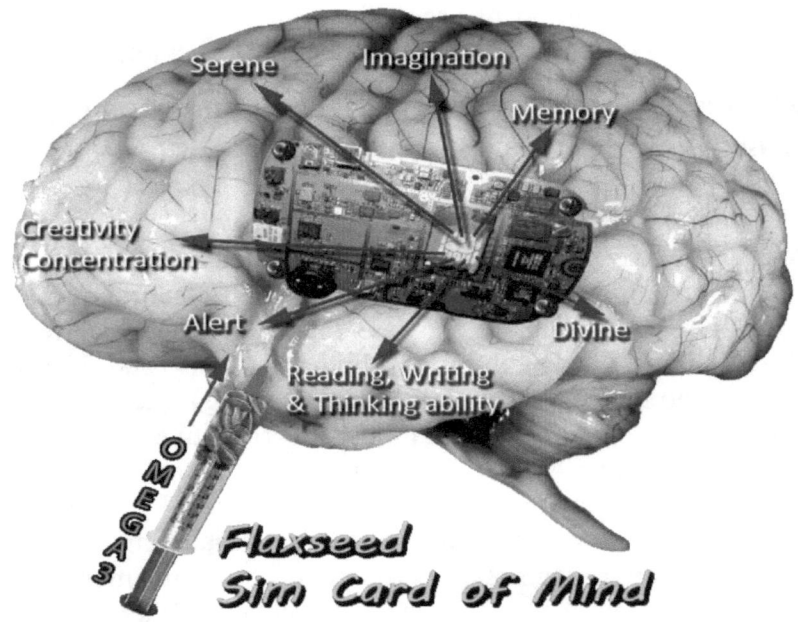

The Flaxseed is a feel good food, keeps your mind cool and you stay cheerful. Negative thoughts stay far away from you. You don't become angry. Your mood is always elated and positive. This is super anti depressant. Studies showed that it improves hostility and criminal behavior in early teens prisoners. Flaxseeds are essential for the function and structure of the brain, improve cognition, memory learning skill and concentration. Flaxseed is SIM CARD of mind's circuit (Mnemonic of flaxseed benefits on mind). Here SIM means Serene, Imagination & Memory and CARD denotes Creativity & Concentration, Alertness, Reading writing & thinking ability and divine. Flax has been scientifically proven to treat depression, diabetic neuropathy, ADHD, Alzheimer's disease, Parkinson's disease, multiple sclerosis and proven to improve the behavior of

Schizophrenics. Flaxseed can improve eyesight and perception of colors. Colors look bolder and vivid. Life becomes simply more colorful.

Choline - Foundation Stone Of Memory

Choline is a water soluble essential nutrient that has extreme importance for the health of cell membranes specially in nervous system. It is an essential part of every person's diet because it is the precursor for the neurotransmitter acetylcholine. This neurotransmitter is responsible for memory and muscle control. Although the body synthesizes some of the choline that it needs, the diet provides the substantial amount 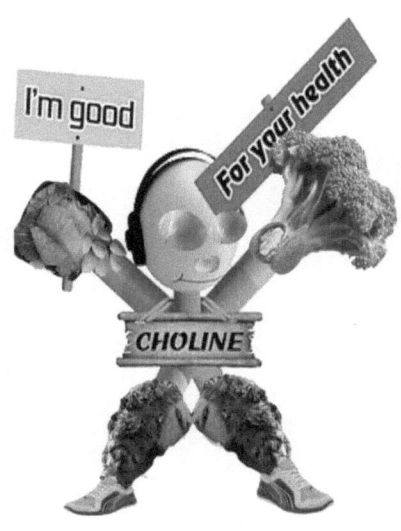 required for health. In the Brain Acetylcholine is the main neurotransmitter for Memory. Its Deficiency directly affects memory. Choline makes Acetylcholine in the brain with the help of Vitamin B-1, B-5, B-12 and Vitamin C. Important sources of Choline are organ meat, eggs, dry fruits, broccoli, chicken, salmon and soybean. The picture shows food sources of choline.

Choline helps memory and brain.

Researchers at Duke University Medical Center found that when they gave choline to pregnant mice their babies had intelligent, developed and much larger brain. Their intelligence, memory and ability to learn has been very good during the entire life. This proves that the choline has capacity to increase memory, learning curve and intelligence. If Choline is given to young persons in sufficient amount, their memory is increases.

In University of Florence Seaford 500 mg of choline was given to 41 people for 5 weeks. Researchers found that their intelligence, wisdom, academic proficiency and memory was increased too much. They also noted that if the choline is given with other memory-enhancing substances e.g. Pyraglutamate they get the full benefit at lesser doses. Choline is essential for construction and maintenance of nerve cell, its covering and neuro-transmitters.

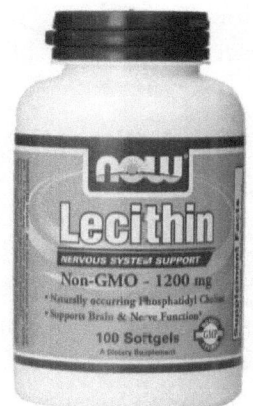

At Massachusetts Institute of Technology Dr. Richard Wartmen said that medications that increase the production of the acetylcholine like piracetam should always be taken with choline otherwise whole choline is spent in the producing acetylcholine and production of nerve cells is interrupted due to this choline deficiency.

Phosphatidyl choline or PC, which is found in Lecithin can cross blood brain barrier easily. Pure choline is full of fishy smell but lecithin is odorless, so people prefer to use Lecithin. Lecithin grains and capsules are easily available at drug stores.

Types and Sources of Choline

There are many types of choline that your body can utilize as a precursor for acetylcholine production. Each has varying strength and advantages / disadvantages. Understanding the interaction between each choline type can influence your diet and other decisions.

Lecithin

This source of choline is one of the most common yet least impactful. Foods like eggs and soy products are filled with lecithin. Even processed foods like chocolate have lecithin added, but choline content is low. As the weakest form of choline, lecithin may not provide enhanced cognitive abilities or prevent neuro degeneration similar to other sources. Supplementing with lecithin typically requires higher dosages to significantly increase acetylcholine levels.

Citicholine (CDP-Choline)

CDP-choline is a more efficient source for providing the acetylcholine precursor. Alone, the CDP-choline has showed great efficacy in solving cognitive decline in elderly patients with Alzheimer's disease. The neuroprotective actions of CDP-choline, along with the ease of passing the blood-brain barrier, makes this an efficient source of choline. Improved learning and memory, along with increased noradrenaline and dopamine levels, make CDP-choline a useful / powerful supplementation for brain health.

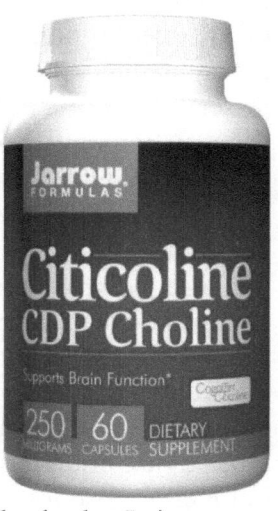

Citicholine is converted to choline in the body. It increases levels of Dopamine and other transmitters. It is often used in the treatment of head injury and stroke because it protects brain from poor blood supply. It also increases memory and learning ability.

L-Alpha Glycerylphosphorylcholine (Alpha GPC)

The Alpha GPC form of choline is one of the most potent. It can be found in the brain and in dairy products, but is typically produced synthetically by purifying soy lecithin. Like, CDP-choline, daily supplementation of Alpha GPC need not be high. It is used to enhance memory and learning for Alzheimer's and dementia patients.

Choline Bitartrate

The choline bitartrate "choline salts" are one of the cheapest sources of choline. It is a weaker choline source than CDP-choline or Alpha GPC, but still provides effective cognitive enhancement if dosed properly.

Dose

- Choline Chloride 500 mg/day
- Lecithin 5-10 gms (1 tbsp/day)
- Phosphatydil Choline 1-2 gms/day
- Citicholine 500-1000 mg/day

Vinpocetine

Vinpocetine is a chemical substance found in the periwinkle plant Vinca minor. People use it as medicine. Because some people think vinpocetine might improve blood flow to the brain, it is used for enhancing memory, cognetion and preventing Alzheimer's disease and

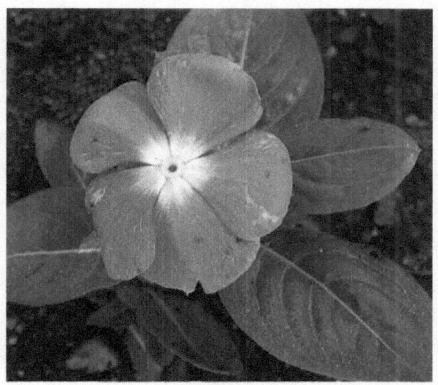

other conditions that harm learning, memory, and information processing skills as people age. It is available in 5 and 10 mg tablets, average dose is 5 mg twice a day.

Ginkgo biloba

Ginkgo biloba, also known as the maidenhair tree, is one of the oldest species of trees on the planet. Ginkgo trees have very unique properties - they are capable of growing more than 130 feet and can live for over one thousand years. In fact, there are some trees in China are said to be over 2,500 years old.

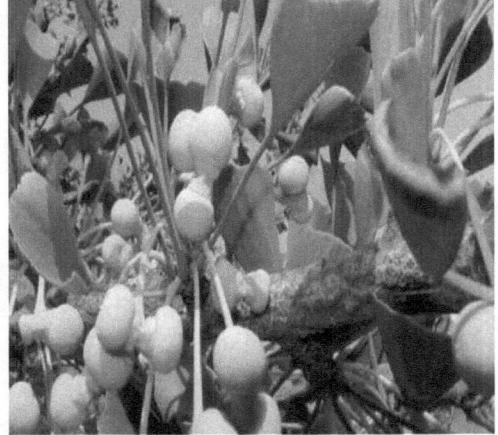

Ginkgo increases concentration of mind and elevates mood. It helps in memory disorder, depression, poor circulation and thinking. The plant has a number of therapeutic properties and contains high levels of flavonoids and terpenoids; these are antioxidants that provide protection against oxidative cell damage from harmful free radicals. Ginkgo helps in production of neurotransmitters and keeps the receptor site of acetylcholine active and healthy. It simply enhances supply of oxygen and nutrients in brain. Experiments have proven that it helps in circulatory defects, memory, concentration, mood and lack of energy.

It is available in 40, 60 and 80 mg capsules. Average daily dose is 120-180 mg means 1 or 2 capsules of 60 mg may be taken twice a day. Effects of ginkgo comes in one or two months. If you do not get desired result in specified period dose may be increased to 240 mg per day. As it is a blood thinner, so vasodilators like aspirin, heparin or coumadin are used with caution.

D.M.A.E.   Dimethyl Amino Ethanol

Sardine is the best source of D.M.A.E. It crosses blood brain barrier and quickly enters the brain. It increases intelligence and memory in the brain.

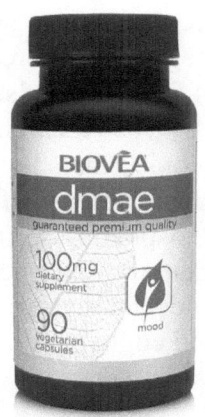

D.M.A.E. increases production of acetylcholine in the brain, reduces stress, increases concentration and learning ability. It also enhances mood and keeps brain alert, energetic and excited.

To increase memory dose of D.M.A.E. is 100-300 mg per day, take in the morning or afternoon but not in the evening. It takes 2 to 3 weeks to get the effect. But the waiting is worth giving very good results.

Phosphatidylserine or "memory molecule"

Phosphatidylserine is also known as "memory molecule". It's literally fills spirit, energy and excitement in the brain. energy and passion that heals. It belongs to phospholipid family and is very important for immunity and the health of liver, nerves and brain.

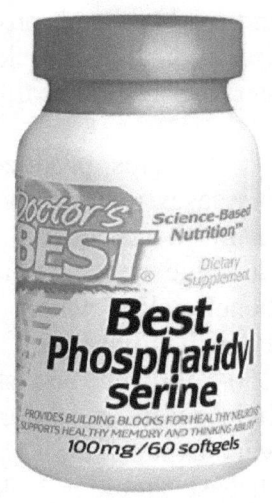

There has been lot of research on Phosphatidylserine and researchers conclude that it is abundant in the brain and increases memory, mood, learning ability, stress-management skills and concentration. It enhances communication, coordination and collaboration between the various tissues of the brain. It is essential component of external coating of nerves and receptor sites of acetylcholine.

It is produced in our body, but this amount is not sufficient. So we have depend on external dietary sources. Its main sources are organ meat specially liver (we may get up to 50 mg per day). Vegetarian sources can hardly provide 10 mg per day. Daily dose of Phosphatidylserine is 100-300 mg a day.

The researchers found that if the diet low in DHA is given to people, then level of Phosphatidylserine becomes very low in hippocampus of brain, which is the center of memory. If Phosphatidylserine is prescribed to dementia patient, it increases memory and cognetion. This means that DHA increases Phosphatidylserine level in hippocampus and it boosts memory and cognetion too much.

Acetyl-L-Carnitine - excellent brain fuel

Acetyl-L-Carnitine is an excellent brain fuel. Its acetyl component helps in production of acetylcholine. It is a potent antioxidant. and protects brain from free-radicals and keeps the entire nervous system healthy and young.

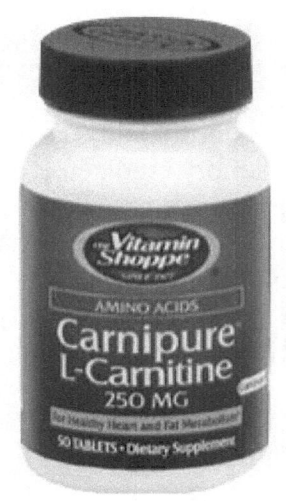

It helps produce new cells and increases interaction between the two hemispheres of the brain, maintains dialogue and cooperation. It is more beneficial when taken with Phosphatidylserine. Its daily doses is 250-1500 mg, and should be taken 1 hour before or 1 hour after meals. It is very expensive and patients of diabetes, liver disease or kidney disease should not take this.

Glutamine - brain fuel

Glutamine is an amino acid which acts as fuel for the brain directly. Glutamine makes the brain more active and keeps you away from any addiction. It helps in production of GABA and glutamate neurotransmitters. It is memory booster. Average daily dose is 2-5 grams per day, you should take it 1 hour prior or 1 hour after meals.

Pyroglutamate and Phosphatidylserine

The transmission capacity of neurotransmitters depend upon proper functioning and active receptor sites. Two nutrients Phosphatidylserine and DHA are very important to keep receptor sites active and functioning. Pyroglutamate enhances number and sensitivity of receptor sites. And thus they boost memory, leaning curve and intelligence.

Pyroglutamate - Minister of information and broadcasting

Pyroglutamate is an amino acid which is found in brain and cerebrospinal fluid abundantly. It boosts memory and all brain powers. It is so effective that medicines derived from this family are highly effective in Alzheimer's Disease; most common symptoms are weak memory and learning disability. Piracetam - derivative of Pyroglutamate is highly researched drug and researchers conclude that it not only boosts memory and learning in patients of memory disorders but also improves memory, learning and intelligence in normal people.

Functions of Pyroglutamate

- Helps in production of acetylcholine
- Increases number of receptor sites of acetylcholine

31

- It increases interaction, dialogue and cooperation between the two hemispheres of the brain. And boosts memory, cognetion, learning and concentration, that means you just become more intelligent and smart
- Main source of Pyroglutamate is fish, milk, curd, butter and vegetables.

Vitamin B Group - Brain Friendly

B Group Vitamins are essential for the brain function. They increase the oxygen supply to the brain and protect from harmful free-radicals. Vitamin B group helps cells make glucose for energy, increase cognition and helps production of neurotransmitters. They are brain's best friends. Let us see how they prove this friendship.

Vitamin B1 (Thiamine)

Thiamine helps whole nervous system to remain fit and fine. It helps brain to produce glucose from carbohydrates for energy. The sources of Thiamine are milk, wheat bran, rice, lentils, chicken, fish, organ meat etc.

Vitamin B3 (Niacin)

It Improves memory. In a study people of different ages were given 141 mg of Niacin per day. people of different ages in the research. There was 10-40% increase in the memory of people of all ages.

Vitamin B-5 Pantothenic acid

It increases mental alertness and memory. It helps in production of acetylcholine. Daily dose for memory benefits is 250-500.

Vitamin B-6 (Pyridoxine)

It helps in production of neurotransmitters by converting amino acids into serotonin, a potent neurotransmitter. Deficiency of serotonin is closely related to depression and several mantel diseases. Daily dose of 20-100 mg is enough to sharpen the memory.

Vitamin B-12 (Cyanocobalamin)

Vitamin B12 improves cognetion and metabolism of fatty acids. It helps in production of Red Blood Cells and makes external insulation coating called myelin sheath of nerve and neurones. Thus Vitamin B-12 keeps our nerves healthy and active. Deficiency of Vitamin B-12 is the main cause of mental weakness, confusion and stupor in old age. Generally, the daily dose is 10-100 microgram. but in old age and certain diseases 1000 micrograms per day is usually prescribed.

Folic acid

Increases oxygen supply to the brain. The daily intake is 400 micrograms.

Brain damaging foods

Today we want to warn you that some foods are very harmful and injurious to both your mind and body, though these are very delicious, attractive, colorful and tempting. Remember these dangerous and killing food items will take you into the deep trench of disaster and trough of failure. You have to quit these if you want high class education, top salary package and success in your life. Isn't leaving a burger and coke worth it.

Alcohol and drugs will certainly damage your brain. Consumption of high "glycemic index" foods, such as bread, burgers, pizza, pasta, cakes, pastries, cookies and sweets cause heavy fluctuation in sugar levels. So the brain gets tired and irritable. Heart clogging fast food and junk food prepared with damaging refined oils reduce blood flow to the brain and is very harmful for mental health. You will avoid the following harmful foods completely.

- Trans fat and Hydrogenated fat including Refined Oil
- Liquor
- Artificial colors and preservatives
- Artificial sugars such as aspartame (Sugar Free) etc.
- Carbonated Drinks
- Sweet beverages
- Bakery products made from refined flour
- Smoking and chewing tobacco

Flaxseed - Miraculous Anti-ageing Divine Food

What is Flaxseed and how can it benefit me? I was thinking about this question when I started hearing about Flaxseed not very long ago. Flaxseed is a 'buzz word' worldwide and seems to be making great role in increased health for many. I wanted to travel in this wagon of wellness and so I researched until I felt satisfied that it could help me, too. These are my findings.

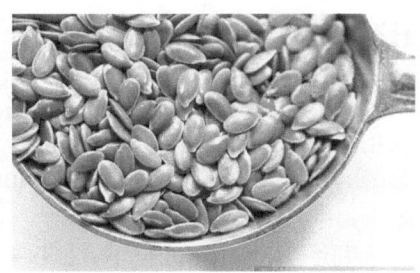

Flaxseed is slightly larger than sesame seed and has a hard shell that is smooth and shiny. The color ranges from deep amber to reddish brown depending upon whether the flax is of the golden or brown variety. The cup-shaped annual, flax flower begins blooming in December and will continue through February, producing abundant blue flowers. Flax plant may reach a height two feet or more at maturity. Botanical name of flaxseed is Linum usitatissimum, which has been widely used for thousands of years as a source of food, clothing and decorating houses (paints, varnish, linoleum flooring etc.). Usitatissimum means useful seeds. The plant's common name, flax, is Middle English, originally from the Old English fleax, and related to the German flachs that means to plait, or interweave, such as in braiding.

The crushed seeds make a very useful poultice used in the treatment of ulceration, abscesses, deep-seated inflammations and even skin cancers.

Flaxseeds have become very popular recently, because they are a richest source of the Omega 3 essential fatty acid; known as Alpha Linolenic Acid (ALA), fiber and lignans a phytoestrogen.

People in the new millennium may see flaxseed as an important food super star.

Flaxseed increase oxygen consumption at the cellular level resulting in increased energy, vitality, stamina and feeling of well-being. In fact, there's nobody who won't benefit by adding flaxseed to his or her diet. It benefits from head to toe and from cradle to grave.

History

Archeological remains indicate that several plants were first cultivated about the same time in Mesopotamia before traveling southward to Egypt. These plants included flax, wheat, barley, peas, lentils and chickpeas.

The Babylonians have been the earliest people to cultivate flax as a food. Linen was used to wrap the mummies of ancient Egypt dating back at least 5,000 BCE. In his epic poem The Iliad (8th century BCE) Homer writes that linen was used for cord and sail-cloth, an indication that the Greeks were cultivating flax plants and were also consuming the seeds. Linen was the fabric used in garments worn by Jewish High Priests. The curtains of the tabernacle were woven of linen.

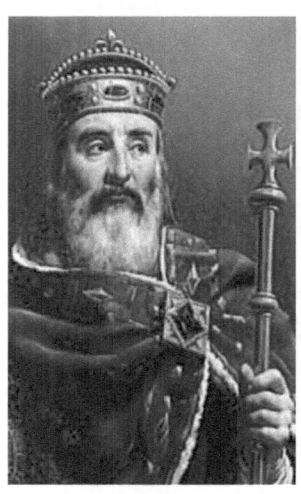

Hippocrates (460 to 377 BCE), a Greek physician who is called the "Father of Medicine," recognized the value of flax in relieving numerous intestinal disorders. When he prescribed flax, his patients benefited from its healing properties.

Charlemagne, the 8th century King of France, regarded flax so highly for its health benefits that he made detailed entries in his medical law books that pertained to the cultivation and use of flax as food and medicine. He ordered his people to consume flax to maintain health and prevent disease (Ragner).

During the middle Ages, the flax flowers were believed to be a protection against sorcery. The Bohemians, who occupied the area that is now Prague, had a belief that centered on seven-year-old children. Families brought their 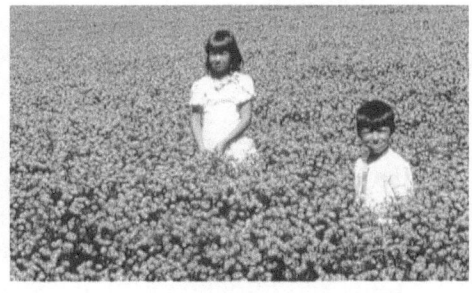 children to dance among the flax fields because their faith that ritual would make the children beautiful. The ritual also recognized that the entire field was under the protection of a Teuton mythological goddess named Hulda, who is said to have passed on her art of growing, spinning, and weaving the flax to mortals (Paradise).

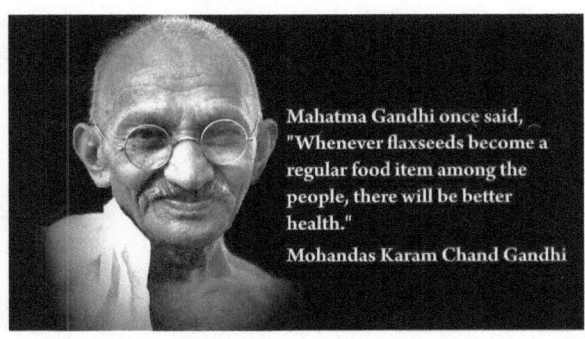

Mahatma Gandhi once said, "Whenever flaxseeds become a regular food item among the people, there will be better health."

Mohandas Karam Chand Gandhi

Flaxseed was grown in India for centuries and was consumed as a oil, food and clothing. Mahatma Gandhi once wrote in a book , "Whenever flaxseeds become a regular food item among the people, there will be a better health (American Nutrition Association, 1972)."

By the 16th century flax cultivation for linen production was a growing industry that brought wealth to local farmers. During this period flaxseeds were consumed as a common food source throughout Europe. Germans, especially, were incorporating them into a variety of whole-grain breads.

Today, flax is grown in Canada and the northern areas of Europe as an alternative crop. The flaxseed has become popular among health conscious Europeans and are readily available in health food stores

Ancient Uses of Flaxseeds and Oil

Linseed oil has long been highly favored oil applied to wooden furniture. Customers were advised to purchase linseed oil at the hardware store and polish the teakwood with it about once or twice a year. It was a custom among farmers to coat their farm tools and implements with flaxseed oil to prevent rust.

After the oil is pressed from the flaxseeds, the remaining cake was sold to farmers as cattle feed. A mixture of honey and flaxseed oil was used as a remedy for removing unwanted spots on the face.

Linseed oil was incorporated as an emollient in making soap and as a drying agent in manufacturing printer's ink, artist's paints, and house paints. The linseed oil is also used in the commercial production of liniments for burns and joint pain. Many farmers regularly feed their animals with flaxseeds to prevent as well as treat diseases.

Making of Flax Oil

A special, cold-pressed and controlled expeller process that does not exceed temperatures of 96^0 F (36^0 C) in order to prevent damage produces truly high quality flax oil. Flax Oil spoils at 42^0 Celsius. Quality flax oil is easily recognized by its lack of odor and its delicate, almost flavorless taste. Some describe the taste of flaxseed oil as slightly nutty. To get the best quality oil the seeds should be organic and pressed only once. After expelling the oil should be packed in dark colored glass bottles with nitrogen flushed. Cold chain should be mentioned during transportation.

You should store the Flax oil in the freeze. You can safely use the oil for four months if you store it in refrigerator and for nine months if you keep it in the freezer section. But at room temperature oil is spoiled in a month. You should also protect the oil from light and air. **The flax oil should never be heated.**

The term expeller pressed involves a mechanical process of pressing the flaxseeds to make oil. Though product labels may say cold pressed, temperatures produced by this process that are not carefully controlled can reach as high as 200^0 F (93^0 C), even though no external heat is applied.

Higher temperatures produce more oil though it is of a lesser quality because flax oil is highly polyunsaturated oil and can easily be damaged by heat, light, and exposure to air. In its damaged state, flax oil becomes tainted with toxic molecules called lipid peroxides that are harmful to the body. The telltale signs are a bitter taste and rancid odor.

Composition of flaxseed

Flaxseed is a highly nutritious food. Flaxseed contains the omega-3 fatty acid, alpha-linolenic acid (ALA), fiber and lignans. About 42% of flaxseed is oil and more than 70% of that oil is comprised of healthy polyunsaturated fatty acids. Flaxseed contains 55-57% of the essential omega-3 fatty acid, ALA.

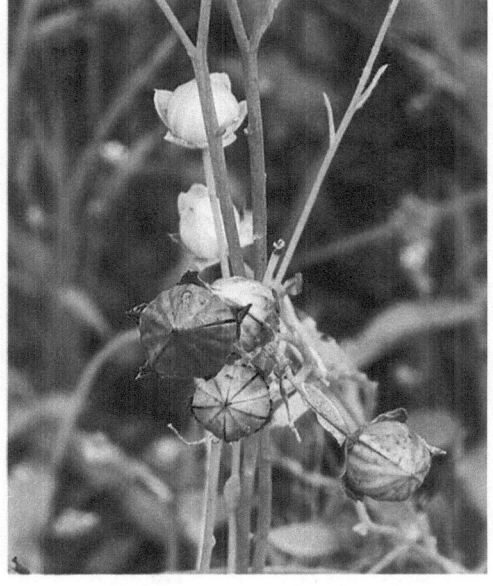

Flaxseed contains soluble as well as insoluble fiber. Soluble fiber can lower blood cholesterol levels and help lower blood sugar, while insoluble fiber moves the stool through the colon more quickly, helping bowel movements and improving evacuation.

Nutrients Name	Nutrient Value	Percentage of RDA
Energy	534 Kcal	27%
Carbohydrates	28.8 g	22%
Protein	18.3 g	32.5%
Total Fat	42.16 g	170%
Dietary Fiber	27.3 g	68%
Vitamins		
Folates	87 µg	22%
Niacin	3.08 mg	19%
Pantothenic acid	0.985 mg	20%
Pyridoxine	0.473 mg	36%
Riboflavin	0.161 mg	12%
Thiamin	1.64 mg	137%
Vitamin C	0.6 mg	1%
Vitamin E	19.95 mg	133%
Vitamin K	4.3 µg	3.5%
Electrolytes		
Sodium	30 mg	2%
Potassium	813 mg	17%
Minerals		
Calcium	255 mg	22.5%
Copper	1.12 mg	124%
Iron	5.73 mg	72%
Magnesium	392 mg	98%
Manganese	2.48 mg	108%
Zinc	4.34 mg	39%
Phyto-utrients		
Lutein-zeaxanthin	651 µg	--

Flaxseed is one of the richest plant sources of lignans, providing up to 800 times more lignans than most other foods. Lignans are phytoestrogens – compounds that have been shown to help protect against certain kinds of cancer, particularly cancers of the breast and colon.

How Linseed became Flaxseed??

Flaxseed oil is now of very popular and used by millions in America for its wonderful health benefits, thanks to two men who fought hard to bring this super oil to U.S.A. Less than 35 years ago, flaxseed was known as "linseed oil." The federal Food and Drug Administration declared that humans shouldn't use it because it was sold as a paint additive.

Mike Minarsich, founder of BioNatures in 1986, read a story about Dr. Johanna Budwig and her amazing work Oil-Protein Cookbook. He wanted to know more, so he searched for the raw, cold-pressed linseed (now flaxseed) oil – at health-food stores and companies. He contacted William Fischer, publisher of Dr. Budwig's book, and discovered that the German publisher had used "edible" linseed oil since he was a child. 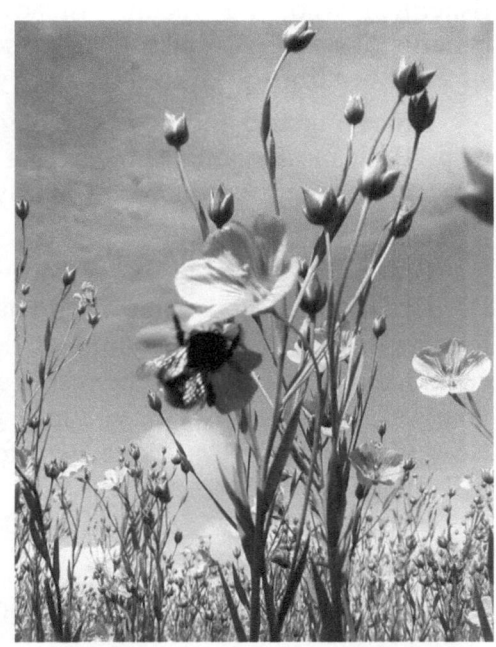 Then, Mike found a Canadian company that produced "linseed" oil according to the standards of Dr. Budwig.

And so he formed BioNatures Company. Bionatures was the first company in America to import and sell linseed oil for human use. Demand soared, in large part because of Fischer's landmark book. But soon the FDA stopped BioNatures' shipments at the Canadian border, claiming that linseed oil is a drying agent for paint and is not suitable for human consumption. BioNatures argued that THIS linseed oil was cold-pressed in a pharmaceutical facility for human consumption and was not the same linseed oil sold in hardware stores. The FDA still said no.

So they came up with two ideas: Find someone in the U.S. to make the product and change the name from linseed oil to flaxseed oil. After all, it was derived from plant that is called the flax plant. Eventually confusion for the government and consumers was eliminated and a partnership established between BioNatures and a young man in northern Washington State named Bruce Barlean and his father. Bruce and his family were fishermen who had vision. Already familiar with the health benefits of omega 3 oils from fish, they saw the potential for the superior benefits of flaxseed oil and byproducts.

Bruce pursued the new idea vigorously. With BioNatures' help, Barleans Organic Oil was born. It is now the country's largest manufacturer, thanks primarily to Bruce and Mike's will power and hard work.

Bruce Barlean made several trips to Germany to visit with Dr. Budwig, developed the proprietary Barlean's Bio-Electron Process TM, used today to produce the oil. It is the only process endorsed by Dr. Budwig. The rest is a history. Today if you type "flax oil" into google.com, you may get around 400,000 results. Now it is considered a staple item for most people's daily diet (Minarsich).

Devotional Song of Goddess Linseed

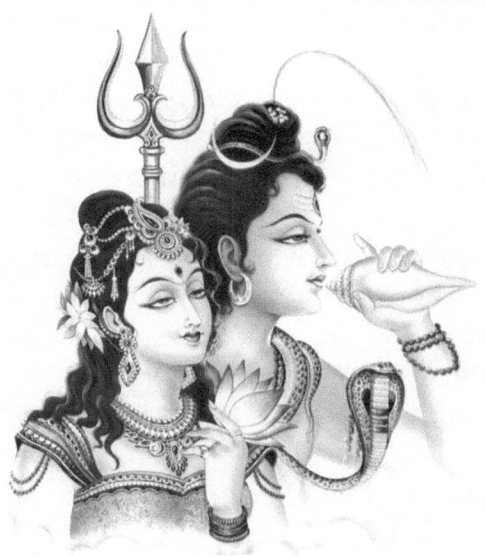

According to Hindu mythology Linseed Goddess is fifth incarnation of Holy Mother Durga. During ancient times Linseed Goddess was worshipped as Scand Mata on fifth day of Navratri festival and linseed was consumed as blessed food (prasad) of Holy Mother. Linseed Goddess is also known as Parvati, Neelpushpi, Kshuma, Uma etc. Linseed is a panacea and balances vata, pitta and kapha all three doshas. The worshipper is blessed with health, vitality and divine power. He never gets sick throughout the year. All of his wishes are fulfilled. Linseed Goddess gives him eternal bliss and straight way opens the door of Moksha (Heaven).

This is a translation of devotion song of Goddess Linseed.

In the Holly books following shloka is written in the praise of Linseed Goddess.

If Lord Shiva and Goddess Parvati are living together, the whole world would be happy and prosperous.

Golden ear pendant and sandal wood cream applied on her forehead is shining like moon.

Master of whole universe holding snake over his body dances with his fair Goddess.

Goddess Linseed is greatest among all other Goddesses, as she keeps everybody healthy and vibrant.

She is a fountain of youth and shines our nails, hair and whole body.

All old Monks say that anger goes away and happiness is achieved.

She supercharges your mind, gives you divine mental powers and flows into the channels of knowledge.

She is an anti-ageing elixir, cures ailments and has unlimited healing properties.

She is symbol of faith, devotion and love. She makes you blissful.

She helps in meditation, arouses your dormant serpent energy (Kundalini) and opens the doors of heaven.

This is the original shloka written ancient Hindu Holy books (Sharma).

अलसी   नीलपुष्पी   पावर्तती   स्यादुमा   क्षुमा।
अलसी   मधुरा   तिक्ता   स्त्रिग्धापाके   कदुर्गरू।।
उष्णा   दृष   शुक   वातंधी   कफ   पित्त   विनाशिनी।

Original Hindi bhajans (Devotional songs) written for Goddess Linseed.

अलसी भजन
शंकर संग सुनंदा भयो रे जग आनंदा
मस्तक चंदन कान के कुंडल चमके जैसे चंदा
गौरा संग नाचे त्रिपुरारी लिपटे देह भुजंगा
सब देवियों में अलसी बड़ी है करदे सबको चंगा
तन में यौवन भर देती है चमके नख शिख अंगा
क्रोध न आए खुशियां लाए कहते सारे महंता
सुमति जगाये सद्गुण आये बहती ज्ञान की गंगा
उम्र बढ़ाये रोग भगाये गुण है तेरे अनंता

44

श्रद्धा भक्ति प्रेम बढ़ाये तू ही परमानंदा
ध्यान लगाये कुंडलि जगाये छूटे जग का फंदा
धुन – नटवर नागर नंदा भजो रे मन..

,,,,,,,,,,,,,,,,,,,,,

अलसी मैया की आरती

आरती अलसी मैया की
शशिधर रूप दुलारी की।।
स्वास्थ्य की देवी कहलाती
भक्त की पीड़ा हर लेती
मोक्ष के द्वार खोल देती
शत्रु हो त्रस्त
रोग हो ध्वस्त
देह हो स्वस्थ
दयामयी उमा सुनीला की
शशिधर रूप दुलारी की।।
त्वचा में लाये कोमलता
कनक जैसी हो सुंदरता
छलकता यौवन का सोता
बदन में महक
केश में चमक
वदन में दमक
मोहिनी नील कुमारी की
शशिधर रूप दुलारी की।।
तुम्हीं हो करुणा का सागर
कृपा से भर दो तुम गागर
धन्य हो जाऊँ मैं पाकर
तू देती शक्ति
करूँ मैं भक्ति
दिला दे मुक्ति
उज्ज्वला मनोहारिणी की
शशिधर रूप दुलारी की।।
ज्ञान और बुद्धि का वर दो
तेज और प्रतिभा से भर दो
'ओम' को दिव्य चक्षु दे दो
न जाऊं भटक
बिछाऊं पलक
दिखादे झलक
रुद्र प्रिय मतिवाहिनी की
शशिधर रूप दुलारी की।।

45

क्रोध मद आलस को हर ले
हृदय को खुशियों से भर दे
आयु और ममता का वर दे
मची   है धूम
मन रहा घूम
भक्त रहे झूम
स्कंद मां पालनहारी की
शशिधर रूप दुलारी की।।
धुन— आरती कुंज बिहारी की

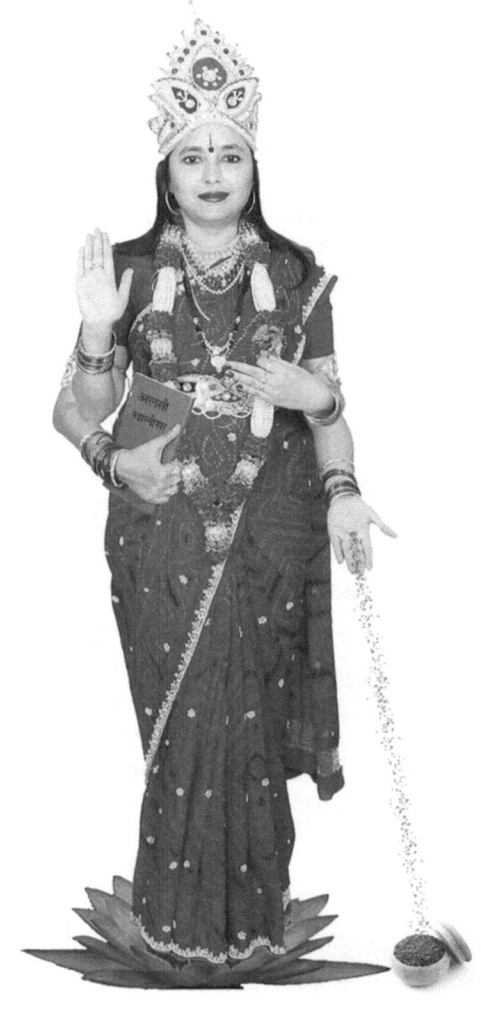

Skin

The skin is the largest organ of the body, with a total area of about 20 square feet. The skin protects us from microbes and external pollutants, helps regulate body temperature, and permits the sensations of touch, heat, and cold.

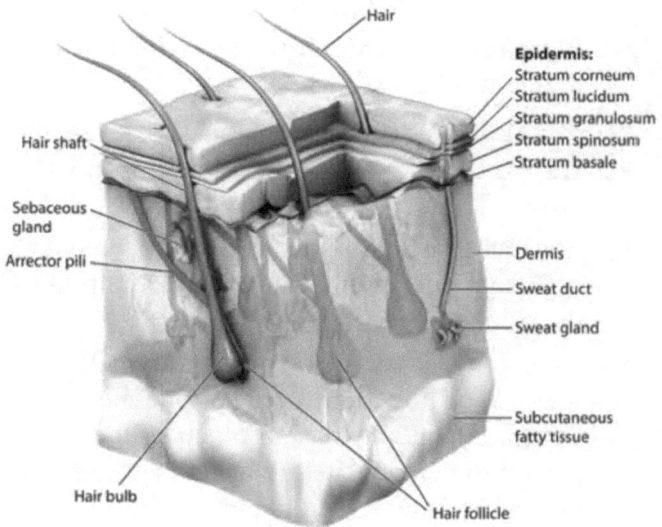

Skin has three layers:

1) **The epidermis on the outside.** This is made from layers of cells with a basal layer, which is always forming new cells through cell division. The new cells gradually move towards the surface, which takes 1-2 months. As they move up they gradually die, become flattened and develop keratin and the outermost layer of flat dead cells is being continually worn away by friction. The keratin and oil from the sebaceous glands help to make the skin waterproof.

2) **The dermis is the inner layer.** The tissues and structures found in the dermis are given below.

- **Elastic fibers** – make the skin resilient.
- **Capillaries** – are tiny blood vessels.
- **Muscle fibers** – to move the position of the hairs.
- **Sensory cells** – to sense touch, pressure, heat, cold and pain.
- **Nerve fibers** – to activate muscles and glands and relay messages from the sensory cells to the brain.
- **Pigment cells which produce Melanin** – a very dark pigment.
- **Sweat glands** which open onto the surface as pores
- **Hair follicles** – pits in the epidermis in which hairs grow.
- **Sebaceous glands** – produce oil to keep hair follicle free from dust and bacteria, and to help to waterproof the skin.
- **There is a layer of fat underneath** and in the lower regions of the dermis. The thickness of this layer varies, depending on the place in the body and from person to person. A store of fat is useful to the body as insulation and it can be used for energy when the intake of nutrients is insufficient.

3) **Connective tissue** – packs and binds the other structures in the skin.

Flaxseed – Skin Healer

If you want one word solution to all your skin, hair and nail problems, my answer is Omega-3 Fats. Free radicals steal electrons from collagen cells in your skin, as a result fine lines are formed in skin which gradually lead to age spots, wrinkles and sagging of skin. Skin becomes dry and looks older. This is ageing of skin.

Omega-3 Key to Healthy skin

Omega-3 fats and Lignans present in flax protect collagen cells and make your skin fair, soft, spotless and charming. Flaxseed is an ultimate edible cosmetic, which glows your skin from inside. It keeps you young and attractive.

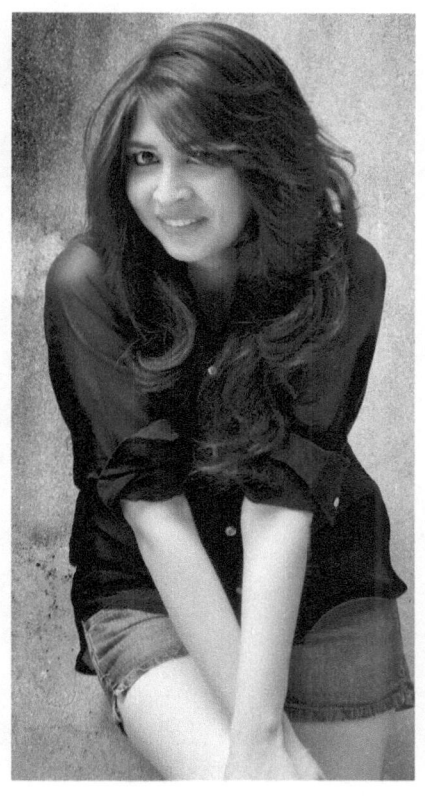

Flaxseed – Skin's best friend

According to Dr. Jeffrey Benabio, dermatologist, Flax protects your skin in two ways. First, everyday irritants are kept from entering skin pores. Secondly, water is locked into your skin when you apply flaxseed oil directly onto your skin. Improving your skin's moisture level can minimize the appearance of wrinkles.

Flaxseed - heals all skin ailments

Flax is full of Omega-3 fats which are Anti-inflammatory and heal inflamed red and itchy skin. These fats also cures skin spots, rashes, ulcers, boils, pimples due to allergy and infection. This way flax treats rosacea, acne, eczema, dandruff, psoriasis and even skin tumors.

Wound healing – Flax oil has been shown to aid in wound healing as well. Wounds heal and recover faster. Possibility of large scar and keloid formation is much less. There is even some evidence that flax oil might protect against ultraviolet light (sun) damage and can help protect you against skin cancer.

Hair

HAIR ANATOMY

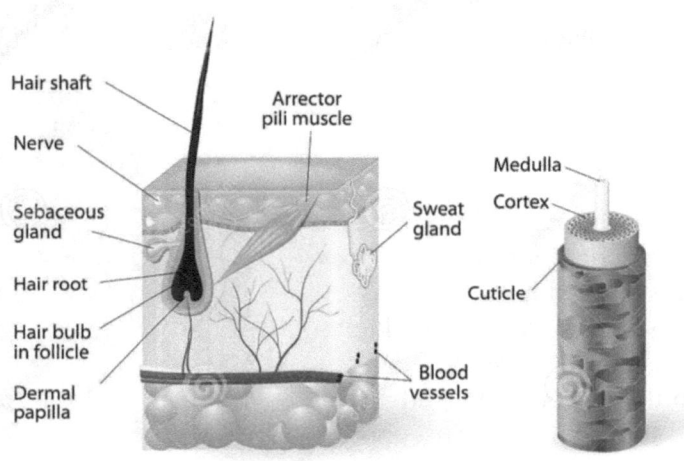

The hair shaft has three layers. Cuticle is the outer transparent layers and gives a shiny appearance to hair. Medulla is the innermost layer composed of large cells. Cortex is the black, thick and hard layer between cuticle and medulla. This contains pigment and keratin.

The root of hair is situated in the skin (epidermis) of scalp. A pouch like structure called follicle surrounds the hair root. Papilla is a large structure at the base of the hair follicle. The papilla is made up mainly of connective tissue and a capillary loop.

Around the papilla is the Matrix, a collection of cells often interspersed with the pigment-producing cells, melanocytes.

Capillaries and nerve fibers indent this bulb. The cells in the center of bulb divide. The newly divided hair cells push the previous cells up. The cells, which move upwards, die slowly forming hard hair shaft.

Each hair grows approximately at the rate of 1 cm per month. This growth continues for 2-6 years. When the hair attains full growth it resets for 2-3 months and is later shed. A new hair starts growing in its place. Thus at any given point of time 10 percent of the total hair on our scalp is in a resting phase and 90 percent of the hair is in growth phase.

Keratin – Building block of Hair

Hair is composed primarily of hard fibrous proteins (88%) known as keratin. It is made in cells of Follicle called keratinocytes, some of these make outer and inner epithelium of follicle, remaining elongate and become shaft of hair. As soon as keratinocyte is filled with keratin, it becomes dead. This way after the growth of 0.5 mm hair becomes mature, dead and does not receive any nutrition afterwards.

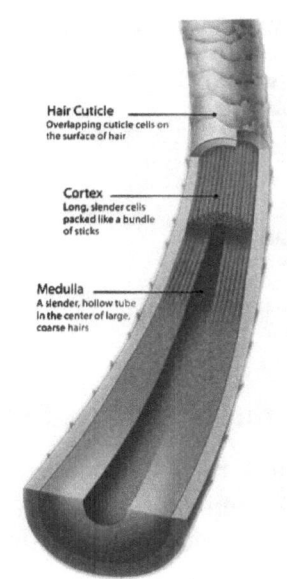

Hair Cuticle
Overlapping cuticle cells on the surface of hair

Cortex
Long, slender cells packed like a bundle of sticks

Medulla
A slender, hollow tube in the center of large, coarse hairs

Sebum - Natural oil of hair and skin

Fats play very important role for strength and shining of hair, even though quantity of fat is just 3%. There are sebaceous glands near hair follicle which produce sebum. It is a mixture of triglycerides, wax and squalene which provide protective coating for skin and hair. And makes skin elastic and shining.

Melanin - Natural Color of skin and hair

Melanocyte cells in the follicle produce natural color pigment Melanin. Keratinocytes take this pigment to give natural color to the hair. There are two main pigments found in human hair: Eumelanin which gives color to brown or black hair and is dark pigment. Pheomelanin is what produces the blonde or red hair.

Flaxseed - Secret of silky hair

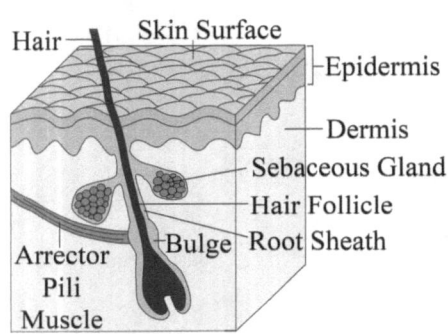

Flax is very miraculous for hair. It is a secret of long, thick, shining, strong and healthy hair. Flax prevent/ reverses premature graying of hair. Lignan has antifungal properties, so regular flax eaters never develop Dandruff.

Essential Nutrients for Hair

Omega-3 Fats - Omega-3 fats are basic building block required to make anti-inflammatory hormones and prostaglandins. They are very essential for healthy scalp skin and sebum production.

Protein – A deficiency can cause you to lose shine and definition, interfere with your moisture levels and ultimately result in stunted hair growth. Sources are whole grains, nuts, beans and legumes, eggs, lean meats, poultry

Vitamin A - Antioxidant that helps produce healthy sebum in the scalp. It's also beneficial to hair follicles, as it keeps the hair root lubricated. Food sources are fish liver oil, liver, meat, milk, cheese, eggs, spinach, broccoli, green leafy vegetables, cabbage, carrots, and orange vegetables, apricots and peaches.

Vitamin B Complex - A deficiency of Vitamin B group may cause hair loss, excessive oil reproduction and premature graying.

Eating things like whole grains, beans and lentils, potatoes and bananas will aid with restoring those deficiencies.

Vitamin C - is what we count on for growth and cell repair. A deficiency can stunt length your hair and interfere with your scalp's circulation and healing abilities. Oranges, papaya, grapefruit, cauliflower and asparagus can help restore depleted levels of Vitamin C.

Vitamin E - plays an important role in proper scalp circulation and the oil levels of your hair strands. A deficiency may cause overly dry, brittle hair and ultimately result in hair loss. Avocados, nuts like almonds and hazelnuts, tomatoes and beets into your diet will help you maintain proper Vitamin E levels.

Silica – Balances calcium and magnesium in the body. It helps to deposit phosphorus in the bones and is vital for strong bones. Silica helps in collagen formation, heals wrinkles, keep skin moist, radiant and young. It is essential for strong, thick, long and lustrous hair. It is also required for nail production. Sources are oatmeal, wheat, rice, millet, onion, beets and green vegetables.

Zinc, selenium manganese and copper – are very important minerals for healthy skin, hair and nails. Deficiency leads to eczema, hair loss and other problems. Zinc reduces levels of DHT which is a major cause of male baldness. Zinc is an anti-oxidant, protects hair Follicle, helps in DNA and RNA production, Reproduction, Growth, Eye and Thyroid Gland functioning. Copper is Anti-inflammatory and is required for healing of wound and wrinkles. It is vital for rich, black and long hair.

Sources of minerals
- Zinc - Spinach, flax, mushrooms, butter, whole grains, legumes, egg, dry fruits etc.
- Selenium – Brazil nut, walnuts, sesame, flax, wheat, soy bean, meat, fish and eggs.
- Copper – Sesame, flax, cocoa, cashew nut, pumpkin and sun flower seeds.

- Manganese – Cloves, red chilies, flax, sesame, dry fruits, cocoa, pumpkin and sun flower seeds.

Biotin – Vitamin of Hair

Biotin or vitamin B7 or vitamin H, supporting the growth of healthy hair, biotin has a direct role in the formation of keratin. It is often prescribed as a treatment for healing dry scalps, treating brittle fingernails and for re-activating hair growth in people experiencing hair loss. It is composed of a ureido ring fused with a tetrahydrothiophene ring. Biotin is a coenzyme for carboxylase enzymes, involved in the synthesis of fatty acids, isoleucine, and valine, and in gluconeogenesis.

It helps cell growth, citric acid cycle, and transport of carbon dioxyde. Sources of biotin are carrot, almonds, walnuts, egg, milk, strawberry, halibut fish, onion, cucumber and cauliflower.

Nail – The Barometer of your health

Our nails are barometer of our general well-being and often act as indicators of health problems elsewhere in the body. It shows status of blood circulation in fingers. Examination of nails help doctor to identify many illnesses or nutrient deficiencies.

Anatomy of Nail

Basically nail is part of skin on the back of finger and toes. And is made of hard and thick protein called keratin. On three sides it is surrounded by skin folds. The hard and visible part of 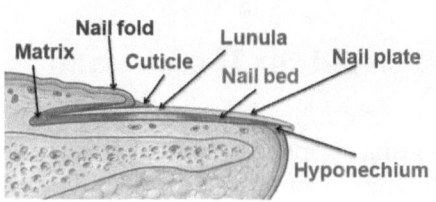 nail is called nail plate. Nail plate is situated and fused over nail bed. The light semicircular proximal part of nail plate is called Lunula. The tissue joining Fold of skin and lunula is called Aponechium or cuticle. Nail grows from matrix situated under the nail cuticle. Nail grows about 0.1 mm in a day.

Nutrients for healthy nails

For making and repair of nails Vitamin B group, Biotin, Calcium, Zinc, Copper, Protein and Omega-3 fats are very important. Their deficiency leads to dry, weak and brittle nails. Vitamin-B deficiency, especially biotin, will 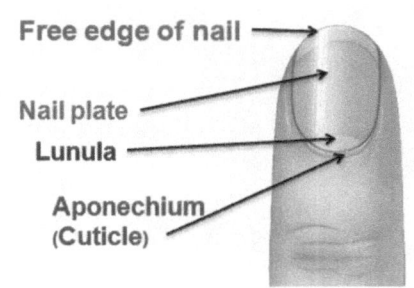 produce ridges along the bed of the nail. Lack of iron causes concave and deformed nails.

Dibutyl Phthalates

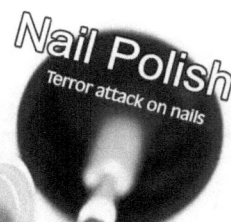

- Affect the function of the central nervous system
- Headaches, fatigue and dizziness.
- Kidney and liver failure.

Toluene

- Wheezing, coughing and irritation to the throat
- Skin irritation and rashes.

Formaldehyde

- Early puberty in girls and uterine problems in women
- Kidney and liver damage
- Birth defects

Flaxseed for Healthy nail

Luckily Flaxseed contains almost all of these nutrients so regular consumption of flaxseed remodels nails and leads to healthy strong, beautiful, pink and spotless nails. Though it does not contain Biotin.

Flax– Good for athletes as well as weight watchers !!!

How is it possible that high-quality cold-pressed flaxseed oil can benefit both top performance athletes to build their lean muscles and obese people who want to get rid of fat deposited in their body? Strange, but it is true. The answer lies in the multiple benefits of alpha-linolenic acid (ALA), found in flaxseed oil in abundance.

Flaxseed oil - great energy source - First, flaxseed oil is a great energy source, especially for endurance athletes and those who burn lots of calories during rigorous workouts. The body does not store enough glycogen to fulfill this energy need. Although the brain uses sugar as its main energy source, the rest of the body uses fat, and flaxseed fatty acids provide clean-burning fuel for tough training routines without disturbing blood sugar level the way refined carbohydrates do.

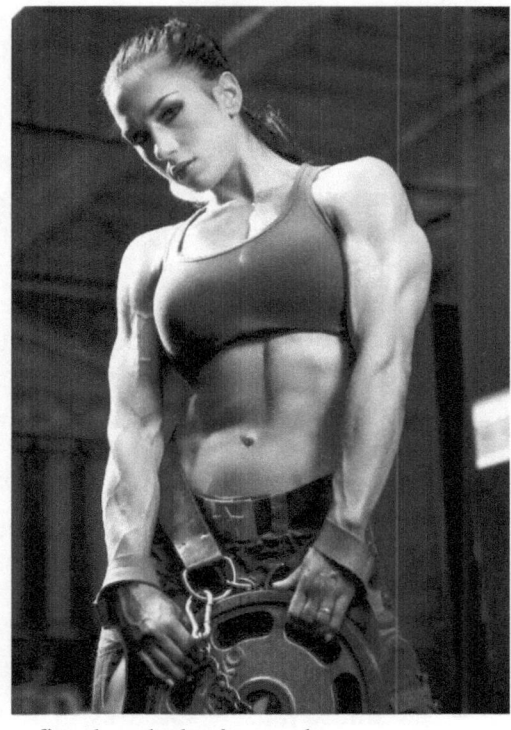

Produce anti-inflammatory molecules Vigorous exercise puts great stress on muscles, tendons, and joint tissues. Fortunately, the local hormones (prostaglandins) synthesized from omega-3 fatty acids (such as EPA produced from ALA) on

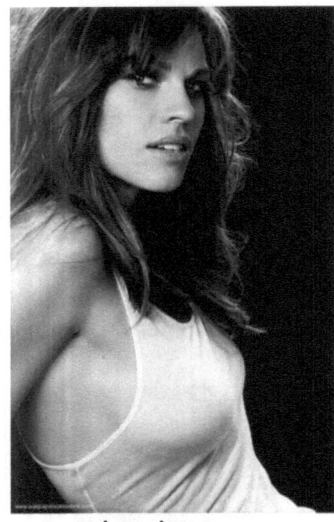

cell membranes are anti-inflammatory. Therefore, the tendency for tissue to become inflamed after exercise is vastly reduced. This benefit shortens recovery time and allows athletes to stay at their performance peak longer.

Make healthy membranes for muscle repair - Vigorous exercise often causes micro-tears in muscles. Protein helps repair muscle cells and essential fatty acids are most important to build cell, nuclear, and mitochondrial membranes that help to remodel and refurbish muscle and connective tissues.

Minimized deposit of subcutaneous fats - For body builders trying to create muscle mass that they want to be seen, the last thing they need is an energy source that will deposit body fat over muscles. This will hide the muscle they have worked so hard to build. Research has demonstrated that animal fats in the diet cause more storage of depot fat on the body than vegetable fats. And of the vegetable fats, ALA sources, such as flaxseed oil, cause the least amount of new fat storage compared to the omega-6 sources, such as corn, sunflower, or safflower oils.

What does all of this mean for **athletes and bodybuilders?**
- Reduced Body fat
- Enhanced Performance
- Shortened recovery time
- Good source of energy
- Reduced muscle soreness
- Increased utilization of oxygen
- Increased utilization of other nutrients
- Overall better health

and what do all of these lead to?   MORE MUSCLE!

The biggest and more publicly discussed example of the benefits of flaxseed oil for athletic performance is preparing Hilary Swank for her role as a boxer in Clint Eastwood's famous film, Million Dollar Baby. A renowned Canadian trainer, Grant Roberts, who owns many gyms in the U.S. and Canada, was given this job. He had the responsibility of adding 10 pounds of lean muscle to her already lean physique in just nine weeks. To everybody's surprise, Mr. Roberts's and Swank's hard work added more than 20 pounds of muscle in that time. How could this be achieved?

An intense weight-training program and lots of practice honing her boxing skills, he put her on a daily 4,000 calorie diet. Half of those calories were in the form of high-protein. One quarter (1000 calorie) of her diet was in the form of flaxseed oil (8 or 9 tablespoons oil in a day). The choice of flaxseed oil was a smart decision based on his hard-earned experience. The film was a big hit 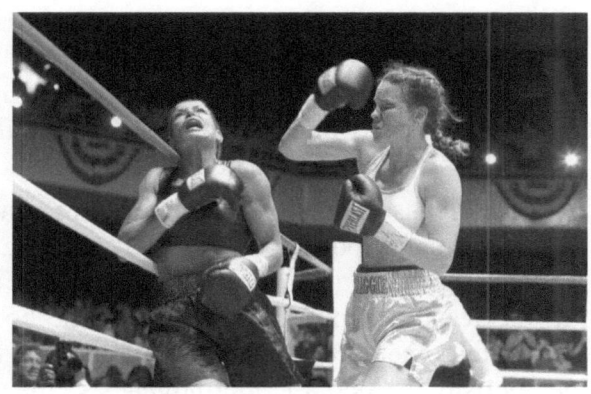 and snatched four Oscar awards.

According to Mr. Roberts, nutrition represents 60% to 70% of the effective input to building lean muscle mass. The remaining 30% to 40% of positive results arise from a wisely planned exercise routine. Thus, there is no substitute for proper nutrition in athletics, and too few coaches and trainers tell this wisdom to their clients.

So why is a top personal trainer like Grant Roberts so keen on using flaxseed oil? In addition to optimal hydration, energy source, flaxseed oil can give a winning shape to the professional or amateur athlete. The benefits of flax oil are wide ranging.

Flaxseed has received an overwhelming response from the athletic and bodybuilding community. An article entitled "Best of the Best", published in the bodybuilding and health enthusiast magazine Muscle Media 2000, claims flaxseed as "the hottest idea in bodybuilding" and "a surprising new category of bodybuilding supplement." Mr. Dan Duchene in his column "Ask the Guru", also writing for Muscle Media 2000, and ranked flaxseed as the number one bodybuilding supplement compared to all other available products.

How does flaxseed oil helps lose Weight

So how do all these benefits of flaxseed oil help to lose weight? First we need to come out of the fat phobia that has been infused in our mind by American media for years. Scientific researchers are now investigating the importance of the type of fat, rather than the absolute quantity of fat, we consume. There are good fats and bad fats. Bad fat is a major risk factor in chronic diseases, while good fats are essential and very important for us. This also applies to obesity and weight management.

Americans normally consume more omega-6 laden animal fats, put more depot fat on the body than natural vegetable oils. And among the vegetable oils, ALA sources, such as flaxseed oil, put the least amount of depot fat on the body. Recent research shows that omega-3 fatty acids actually help to enhance the body metabolism to increase thermogenesis, the generation of body heat to burn off excess calories.

Sprouting flaxseeds

Making sprouts of flaxseeds is so easy you won't believe it! They just can't be done any other way... otherwise these become too gelatinous and spoil. Just put the seeds directly on a steel plate and watch them grow!

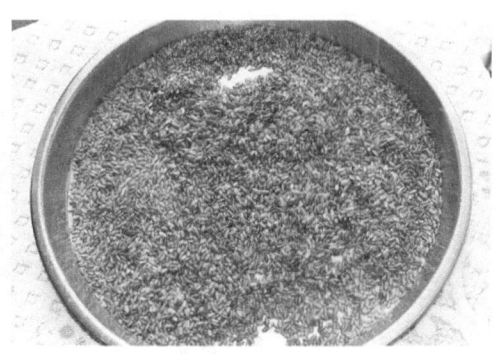

You need the following items.

- Two large stainless steel plates
- Water spray bottle
- Flaxseeds approx 100 grams

Procedure – Take a stainless steel plate and spread the flaxseeds evenly in this plate. Then fill RO water in the spray bottle. Nicely spray water over flaxseeds. Cover this plate with another steel plate and keep these on a table. After 15 minutes

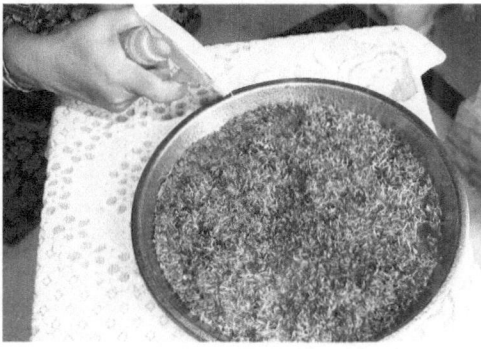

remove the cover plate and check the flaxseeds in the bottom plate. You will see that flaxseeds have absorbed all the water and are almost dry. Spray the water over flaxseeds again, cover and keep upon the table. In the beginning check the flaxseeds frequently and spray water if desired. Afterwards it is enough to check every 3-4 hours in a day. The basic idea is that you give controlled amount of moisture to the seeds. If you pour more water, the soluble fiber mucilage swells up and become gelatinous. If everything is fine, you will get beautiful flaxseed sprouts on third day. Sprouts may have approx. 1 cm. long white and shining roots. We have tried many procedures, but this is the best procedure to make wonderful flax sprouts.

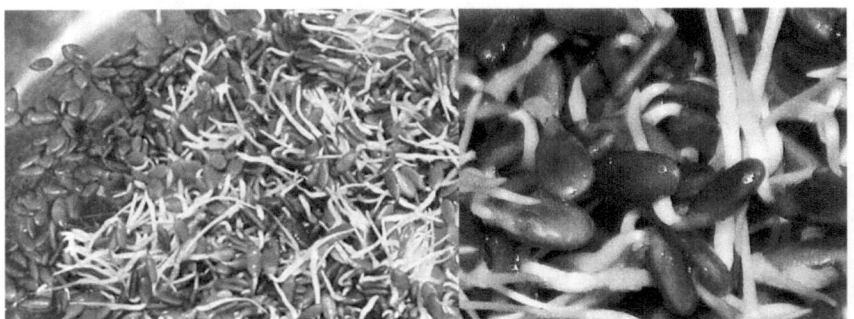

Adding flaxseed to your diet

Flaxseed adds a pleasant, nutty taste to foods. You can buy raw Flaxseed, already ground Flax meal, Flaxseed Oil, or Flax Oil Capsules. Here are some ways to use flaxseed.

- Whole flaxseeds add color and crunch to foods. You can sprinkle flaxseed powder on top of home baking or mix them into a dough.
- Grinding whole seeds breaks their tough outer skin, creating a light-colored powder. Milled flaxseed is sold in a vacuum packs or you can prepare it yourself in a coffee grinder. Sprinkle milled flaxseed on cereal or add it to doughs, batters, casseroles and other cooked foods.
- **Flaxseed oil** is sold in bottles. It is a **sun shine** in a bottle. Pour flaxseed oil on fresh salads. Flaxseed oil provides ALA but no fiber or lignans. Flaxseed oil is also available in gel capsules and sold as a dietary supplement.
- Omega-3 enriched eggs contain extra omega-3 fatty acids from flaxseed fed to hens. You can use omega-3 eggs wherever you would use regular eggs – there's no taste difference, only nutrition enrichment. If eaten on a regular basis, omega-3 enriched eggs make a substantial contribution to your need for omega-3 fatty acids. The caloric value and protein content of omega-3 enriched eggs are similar to that of regular eggs.
- Omega-3 enriched foods, such as yogurt and milk, may contain flaxseed oil, while flaxseed baked goods, such as breads, can include milled or whole flaxseed.
- Whole flaxseeds do not break down in the digestive system. If you consume them whole, chew them thoroughly. Even then, many may not have broken down and will pass through the digestive system without being absorbed. Still, they offer the benefits of fiber by

cleansing the intestinal tract. Store flaxseed meal in the refrigerator.

- Be sure to drink plenty of water when consuming flaxseeds or the flaxseed meal because flax tends to absorb large quantities of liquid during the digestion process.
- Raw is the only way to consume flax oil. Do not use flax oil for cooking. When polyunsaturated oils such as flaxseed oil are subjected to high heat, their chemical make-up is converted to unhealthful lipid peroxides.

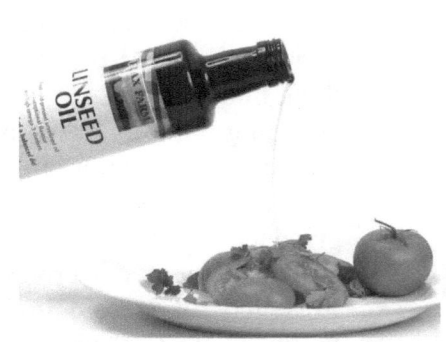

How much flax to eat

- Like any high fiber food, flaxseed may upset your digestion if you add too much, too quickly. Healthy people should consume 15-20 g (2-3 Tbsp.) of milled flaxseed as part of a balanced diet.
- **For individuals at risk of developing, or who have heart disease, a daily intake of 40g (5 Tbsp.) of milled flaxseed is recommended by Health Department of Canada.**

Storing Flaxseed

You can store whole flaxseed, which is clean, dry and of good quality, at room temperature for up to a year.

To keep flaxseed fresh, you should grind it when you need it. You can keep milled flaxseed refrigerated in an airtight, opaque container for up to 30 days, but it is not recommended.

Fat or Oil Substitution Instructions

Use a 3:1 ratio when substituting flaxseed for oil in a recipe. For example, 3 tablespoons of milled flaxseed can replace 1 tablespoon of butter, margarine, shortening or vegetable oil.

Egg Substitution Instructions:

For every egg being replaced, mix 1 tablespoon milled flaxseed with 3 tablespoons water in a small bowl and let sit for one or two minutes. The mixture will become gel-like. Add to your recipe as you would an egg.

Extract of my experience

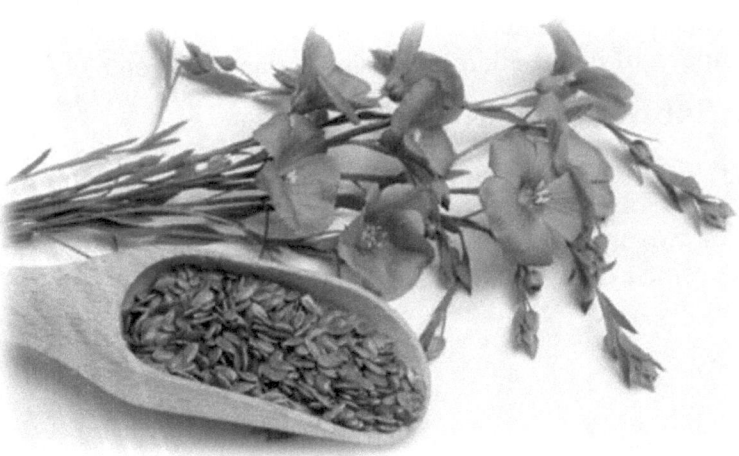

To increase the overall metabolism of the brain, intelligence and memory, we suggest some changes in your diet. You may also take some supplements and medicines. So that you get full benefit of your hard work and you get highest marks in every examination. You will always achieve top ranks and get admission in the desired institution. The most suitable recipe of your success is as follows:

- Consume 20-30 grams of freshly ground Flaxseeds everyday to get enough omega-3 fatty acids required for your brain.
- Fish eaters may ear Omega-3 rich Salmon, Mekrel, herring, Halibut, Sardine etc.
- Eat Vitamin B complex or multivitamin tablet regularly throughout the year.
- You may take at least two supplements mentioned above. Choline is really important. But always consult your doctor before taking any supplement.

My Publications

Awesome Flax: A Book by Flax Guru [Kindle Edition]

http://www.amazon.com/Awesome-Flax-Book-Guru-ebook/dp/B00PUUIR0K

Book Description

Publication Date: November 18, 2014 | Age Level: 1 - 18 | Grade Level: P - 12

Flaxseed- Miraculous Anti-ageing Divine Food

What is Flaxseed and how can it benefit me? I was faced with this question when I started hearing about Flaxseed not long ago. It became a 'buzz word' in society and seems to be making great role in increased health for many. I wanted to join that wagon of wellness and so I researched until I felt satisfied that it could help me, too. Here are my findings.

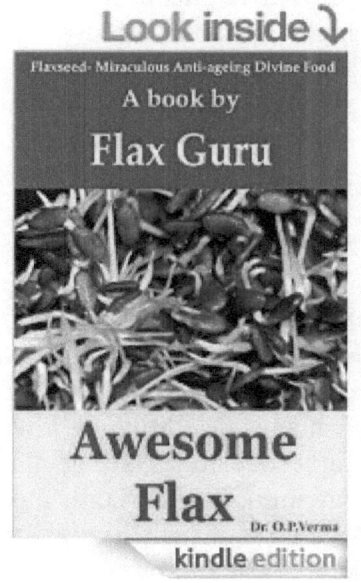

Flaxseeds are the hard, tiny seeds of Linum usitatissimum, the flax plant, which has been widely used for thousands of years as a source of food and clothing. Flaxseeds have become very popular recently, because they are a richest source of the Omega 3 essential fatty acid; also known as Alpha Linolenic Acid (ALA) and lignans. People in the new millennium may see flaxseed as an important new FOOD SUPER STAR. In fact, there's nobody who won't benefit by adding flaxseed to his or her diet. Even Gandhi wrote: "Wherever flaxseed becomes a regular food item among the people, there will be better health."

Flaxseed contains 30-40% oil (including 36-50% alpha linolenic acid, 23-24% linoleic acid- Omega-6 fatty acids and oleic acids), mucilage (6%), protein (25%), Vitamin B group, lecithin, selenium, calcium, folate, magnesium, zinc, iron, carotene, sulfur, potassium, phosphorous, manganese, silicon, copper, nickel, molybdenum, chromium, and cobalt, vitamins A and E and all essential amino acids.

Other fatty acids, omega-6's, is abundant in vegetable oils such as corn, soybean, safflower, and sunflower oils as well as in the many processed foods made from these oils. Omega-6 fatty acids have stimulating, irritating and inflammatory effect while omega-3 fatty acids have calming and soothing effect on our body. Our bodies function best when our diets contain a well-balanced ratio of these fatty acids, meaning 1:1 to 4:1 of omega-6 and omega-3. But we typically eat 10 to 30 times more omega-6's than omega-3's, which is a prescription for trouble. This imbalance puts us at greater risk for a number of serious illnesses, including heart disease, cancer, stroke, and arthritis. As the most abundant plant source of omega-3 fatty acids, flaxseed helps restore balance and lets omega-3's do what they're best at: balancing the immune system, decreasing inflammation, and lowering some of the risk factors for heart disease.

One way that Omega 3 essential fatty acid known as Alpha Linolenic Acid ALA helps the heart is by decreasing the ability of platelets to clump together. Flax seed helps to lower high blood pressure, clears clogged coronaries, lowers high blood cholesterol, bad LDL cholesterol and triglyceride levels and raises good HDL cholesterol. It can relieve the symptoms of Diabetes Mellitus. It lowers blood sugar level. Flaxseed help fight obesity. Adding flaxseed to foods creates a feeling of satiation. Furthermore, flaxseed stokes the metabolic processes in our cells. Much like a furnace, once stoked, the cells generate more heat and burn calories.

Flaxseeds are the most abundant source of lignans. Lignans are plant-based compounds that can block estrogen activity in cells, reducing the risk of Breast, Uterus, Colon and Prostate cancers. According to the US Department of Agriculture, flaxseed contains 27 identifiable cancer preventative compounds. Lignans in flaxseeds are 200 to 800 times more than any other lignan source. Lignans are phytoestrogens, meaning that they are similar to but weaker than the estrogen that a woman's body produces naturally. Therefore, they may also help alleviate menopausal discomforts such as hot flashes and vaginal dryness. They are also antibacterial, antifungal, and antiviral.

Because they are high in dietary fiber, ground flaxseeds can help ease the passage of stools and thus relieve constipation, hemorrhoids and diverticular disease. Taken for inflammatory bowel disease, flaxseed can help to calm inflammation and repair any intestinal tract damage.

Cancer - Cause and Cure: Based on Quantum

Physics developed by Dr. Johanna Budwig

http://www.amazon.com/Cancer-Quantum-Physics-developed-Johanna-ebook/dp/B00P3Y7BYG

Book Description

Publication Date: **October 31, 2014** | Age Level: **10 - 18** | Grade Level: **7 - 12**

***** A must have book for every cancer patient *****

This book provides both an introduction of Dr. Budwig's cancer research and treatment. Johanna Budwig (1908-2003) who was nominated for the Nobel Prize seven times was one of Germany's leading scientists of the 20th Century, a biochemist and Cancer specialist with a special interest in essential fats.

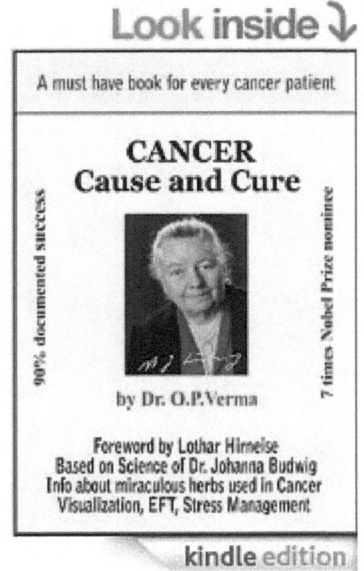

Otto Warburg proved that prime cause of cancer oxygen-deficiency in the cells. In absence of oxygen cells ferment glucose to produce energy, lactic acid is formed as a byproduct of fermentation. He postulated that sulfur containing protein and some unknown fat is required to attract oxygen in the cell.

In 1951 Dr. Budwig developed Paper Chromatography to identify fats. With this technique she proved that electron rich highly unsaturated

Linoleic and Linolenic fatty acids were the undiscovered mysterious decisive fats in respiratory enzyme function that Otto Warburg had been unable to find. She studied the electromagnetic function of pi-electrons of the linolenic acid in the membranes of the microstructure of protoplasm, for all nerve function, secretions, mitosis, as well as cell break-down. This immediately caused lot of excitement in the scientific community. New doors could open in Cancer research. Hydrogenated fats, including all Trans fatty acids were proved as respiratory poisons.

Then Budwig decided to have human trials and gave flaxseed oil and quark to cancer patients. After three months, the patients began to improve in health and strength, the yellow green substance in their blood began to disappear, tumors gradually receded and at the same time the nutrients began to rise. This way Dr. Budwig had found a cure for cancer. It was a great victory and first milestone in the battle against cancer. Her treatment protocol is based on the consumption of flax seed oil with low fat cottage cheese, raw organic diet, mild exercise, and the healing powers of the sun. She treated approx. 2500 cancer patients during a 50 year period with this protocol till her death with over 90% documented success.

She was nominated 7 times for Nobel Prize but with a condition that she will use chemotherapy and radiotherapy with her protocol. They did not want to collapse the 200 billion business over night. She always refused to support the damaging chemo and radio for the sake of humanity.

Lothar Hirneise is founder and President of People Against Cancer, Germany. He travels a lot in search of finding most successful alternative cancer therapies. He has been student of Dr. Johanna Budwig. He is a great researcher and writer on alternative healing. He is successfully treating thousands of cancer patients at his 3-E center in Germany. In the last few years he has interviewed several hundred final stage so-called survivors, meaning patients who were in the final stage of cancer and who are all healthy again today. Based on his findings he proposed a 3 E Program – The Mnemonic of Cancer Treatment.

1) Eat well
2) Eliminate
3) Energy

He noticed that 100% of all survivors, did the energy work. In approximately - say 80% of all patients, He found a change in diet. And in at least 60% of all patients, took intensive detoxification rituals. This is the basis of his, so much talked about 3E Program for healing cancer.

Lothar Hirneise strongly supports holistic and spiritual approach and includes Visualization, Tumor Contract, Meditation, mild Yoga, Emotional Freedom Technique EFT, Dr. Ryke Geerd Hamer's New German Medicine (Connection of unresolved stress and cancer), Detoxification techniques (Soda Bicarb bath, Epsom bath, Sauna, Colon Hydrotherapy, Coffee Enema etc.)in his so much talked about 3 E Program.

The book also, describes about rare and miraculous herbs used in the treatment of Cancer like Turmeric, Black seed, Ginger, Mistle Toe, Aloe vera, , Echinecea, Lobelia, Essiac Tea, Pau d'arco Tea, Dandelion, Milk Thistle

www.ingramcontent.com/pod-product-compliance
Lightning Source LLC
Chambersburg PA
CBHW050508290526
45786CB00006B/2489